Johnny Rockerm

CW00539998

An overview of Cancer as a metabolic disease by Dr. Thomas Seyfried.

Student Edition.

On the Origin, Management, and Prevention of Cancer

Featuring Dr. D'Agostino, Dr. Attia, Dr. Chaffee

Revised Transcripts

(final revision of Chapter 1 - by Dr. Thomas Seyfried)

25% of the royalties will go to cancer research, via
The Foundation for Metabolic Cancer Therapies
See Ketoforcancer.net

ANY REVIEW WOULD BE GREATLY APPRECIATED TO GET THE MESSAGE OUT!

Table of Contents

Chapter 1: Dr. Thomas Seyfried – Cancer as a metabolic disease

Well, thank you very much. I'd like to thank CrossFit and Greg for supporting us. I'd also like to thank Jeff Glassman for the good questions that he asked us in the past, to validate some of our theories. You know, we need people like that, it's good to have people that question the information that you present. It makes us better at explaining this.

For your information: I have no financial disclosures.

Alright, So what I'd like to do to start this off is, basically, to present a report card on our approach to managing cancer.

And as I said, I'm going to speak to you today about cancer in general and also focus on specific types of cancer, in particular glioblastoma. As an illustrative example of our approach to managing the disease.

Now, these are numbers that we can take from the American Cancer Society, and they publish every year data on the overall number of cases and deaths. The war on cancer and the success that we're having is not going well.

So I compiled the data, just over the last five years:

Percentage increase for cancer deaths is greater than the increase for new cases!

Cancer Statistics in the U.S. from 2013-2017

Year	New Cases	Deaths/year	deaths/day
2013	1,660,290	580,350	1,590
2014	1,658,370	585,720	1,605
2015	1,658,370	589,430	1,615
2016	1,685,210	595,690	1,632
2017	1,688,780	600,920	1,646
% Increase	1,7%	3,4%	3,4%

Data from American Cancer Society

This is 2013 to 2017 and as you can see, these are pretty sobering numbers. We break them down into new cases, deaths per year and deaths per day, simply dividing by 365, to give an estimate. And you'll notice that the deaths per day and per year are exceeding that of the new cases. Not good.

Just to put things into perspective: The population increase in the United States over the same period of time was about 2.9 percent. So how is this war on cancer going? You look at the numbers, you can make your own decision. These are numbers you don't see on TV, right? You see Opdivo and Keytruda and that kind of stuff, but you don't see the constant increase in deaths per day.

So the question we have to ask ourselves is: What's going on here? We're not getting success here! This is a failure of monumental proportions, right? These are large numbers! In China it's over 8,000 a day dying from cancer. Cancer's already superseded heart disease in China!

We go out and we raise money for cancer, right? You all know, you run, jump... I don't know if you guys do 'CrossFit for cancer'. But everybody raises money for cancer, it makes them feel good. Nobody asks: How much of the money that we raise goes to cancer research? And what's more important: What kind of research are they doing with all that money?

The federal government's spending millions of dollars on cancer research. People are raising money, "Stand up to cancer!" Look, the more money we raise for cancer, the more cancer we get. So you have to say: What is going on here? How do you explain this?

And it has to do with a fundamental misunderstanding of what the nature of this disease is.

We've been led to believe, that this is a genetic disease and I'll present evidence to show that it's not.

Here's a simple cartoon of a cell with a nucleus and a mitochondrion, within a cell membrane:

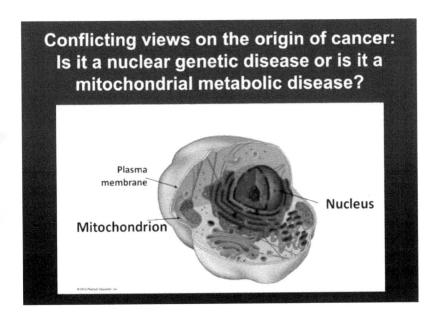

Conflicting views on the origin of cancer: Is it a nuclear genetic disease or is it a mitochondrial metabolic disease?

- Plasma membrane
- Nucleus
- Mitochondrion

So we know there are mutations in the nucleus, but we also know that there are defects in the mitochondria as well. And I'll be showing you data showing that the origin of this disease is a mitochondrial metabolic abnormality. It's not a nuclear genetic disease. The mutations that you see in the nucleus are actually coming from reactive oxygen species (ROS) produced by the mitochondria!

What the entire field has been doing over the last six or seven decades, is chasing red herrings! Consequently, you have 1,600 people a day dying from the disease.

So the current dogma says: **Cancer is a genetic disease**. And this is solidified in this major paper:

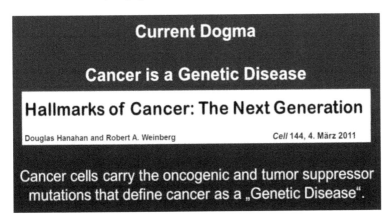

Current Dogma

Cancer is a Genetic Disease

Hallmarks of Cancer: The Next Generation

Douglas Hanahan and Robert A. Weinberg — *Cell* 144, 4. März 2011

Cancer cells carry the oncogenic and tumor suppressor mutations that define cancer as a „Genetic Disease".

Hallmarks of Cancer by Hanahan and Weinberg, one of the more highly cited papers in the entire cancer field. What they say is: Cancer cells carry the oncogenic and tumor suppressor mutations that define cancer as a genetic disease.

And we say it's a dogma, because it's presented as if it is an irrefutable truth. A dogma is no longer questioned, it's a solidified viewpoint. If you go into any textbook of biology, biochemistry or cell biology and you go to the cancer section, it says "cancer is a genetic disease." You go on to the NCI website, the National Cancer Institute, "cancer is a genetic disease."

There's no discussion about anything other than the fact that cancer is a genetic disease. Many of you went to medical school, you probably learned that cancer is a genetic disease. All the college courses on cell biology: Cancer is a genetic disease.

What this concept has done now, is it has indoctrinated several generations of scientists and physicians into this viewpoint that cancer is a genetic disease.

The somatic mutation theory is the foundation upon which the viewpoint of "cancer is a genetic disease" is based. And, basically, what the somatic mutation theory says, is that "Well, we get random mutations":

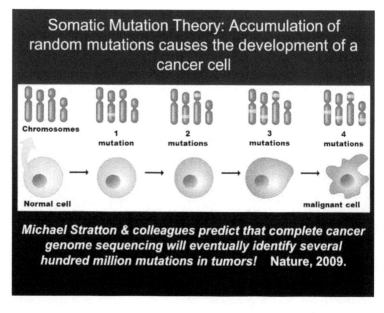

Somatic Mutation Theory: Accumulation of random mutations causes the development of a cancer cell

Chromosomes — Normal cell — 1 mutation — 2 mutations — 3 mutations — 4 mutations — malignant cell

Michael Stratton & colleagues predict that complete cancer genome sequencing will eventually identify several hundred million mutations in tumors! Nature, 2009.

<u>Random</u> mutations that accumulate. And eventually, you convert a normal appearing cell into this dysmorphic, mesenchymal kind of cell.

6

But nobody really knows how many mutations it takes to cause... or how it is related to the formation of a tumor. Is it 1, 2, or 4 mutations?

Michael Stratton from the UK says "We're going to have 100 million genes going to be found," and "look at the deep sequencing coming out of the Broad Institute," and these various places." Thousands and thousands of mutations have been identified.

And then they have to label them with different names, "drivers" and "passengers" and "go-alongs". A whole bunch of stuff is going on there.

And no one talks about those cancers that have no mutations! Kind of non-discussed.

So where does that all lead us to? Where have we come in this journey to manage cancer? We have now come to these terms "personalized therapy", "precision medicine"... all of this is based on the viewpoint that cancer is a genetic disease.

So you have these kinds of images, here:

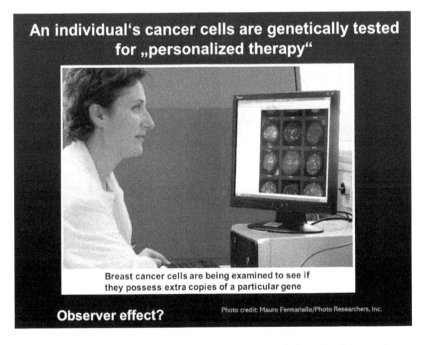

An individual's cancer cells are genetically tested for „personalized therapy"

Breast cancer cells are being examined to see if they possess extra copies of a particular gene

Observer effect?

Photo credit: Mauro Fermariello/Photo Researchers, Inc.

You have this woman staring into a screen and she's looking at breast cancer information to see if this may possess extra copies of a particular gene. Which would be used, in theory, as a diagnostic tool with possibly some therapeutic application. Now, to get that information usually you do needle biopsy.

So you have to take a needle biopsy of a particular tissue, in this case it would be a breast cancer. So you stab the tissue and in the process of stabbing the tissue, to get the information that she's looking at on that screen. Biopsy changes the micro environment of the tissue. You have potentially taken a pre-malignant state and by stabbing it to get this information, you have now put that person at risk.

Now, very interesting: The information that you get for this kind of screening is about $7,200 to do one of these screenings. To get the information that you can look at and say "Oh, we have this kind of battery of genes." Now, this would be okay if it had any redeeming value, right? But it has no value.

But you put people at risk for cancer by the very process of taking tissue. The phenomena is called inflammatory oncotaxis: It's an observer effect. By looking at it, you've changed it.

Now, I want to talk to you about the evidence that does not support the somatic mutation theory of cancer. And whenever you challenge any kind of a solidified dogma you always get the same response. We saw one of these images yesterday. This comes from Nikko, Japan. These are the Nikko monkeys:

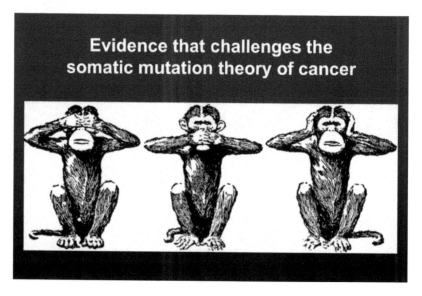

I went to japan, actually. They have carvings of them that are a little bit different than this, but it's basically similar: You don't want to look at the data, you don't want to talk about it, you don't want to hear about it. Anything that challenges your world view. I don't care if it's a religion, a political philosophy or a scientific concept. You generally get this kind of a response. I know it's hard, it's hard for people to look at things differently.

8

So what I did in chapter 11 of my book... This is a paper that I wrote a couple of years after the book, to update more and more of the issues associated with information that does not support the somatic mutation theory:

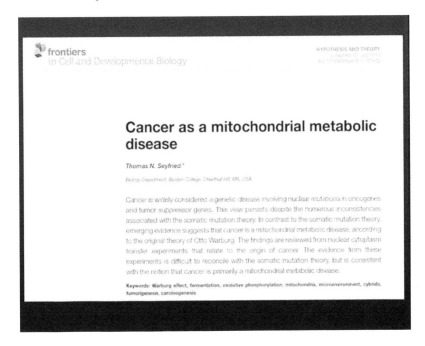

frontiers
in Cell and Developmental Biology

HYPOTHESIS AND THEORY

Cancer as a mitochondrial metabolic disease

Thomas N. Seyfried *

Biology Department, Boston College, Chestnut Hill, MA, USA

Cancer is widely considered a genetic disease involving nuclear mutations in oncogenes and tumor suppressor genes. This view persists despite the numerous inconsistencies associated with the somatic mutation theory. In contrast to the somatic mutation theory, emerging evidence suggests that cancer is a mitochondrial metabolic disease, according to the original theory of Otto Warburg. The findings are reviewed from nuclear cytoplasm transfer experiments that relate to the origin of cancer. The evidence from these experiments is difficult to reconcile with the somatic mutation theory, but is consistent with the notion that cancer is primarily a mitochondrial metabolic disease.

Keywords: Warburg effect, fermentation, oxidative phosphorylation, mitochondria, microenvironment, cybrids, tumorigenesis, carcinogenesis

All I did was take articles from the literature that had been spattered about for years and brought them all together in one group of papers - and reevaluated the information from those papers in light of the two competing theories for the origin of the disease. So, bring them all together and then look at the data and then say "Do the data support more strongly one hypothesis, or theory, over the other?"

And you come to the conclusion that the somatic mutation theory makes no sense,- relative to the mitochondrial metabolic theory. You know, what's very interesting about this, when Gary gave his talk yesterday... about the difficulty in reproducing findings...

I find it remarkable that these different kinds of experiments were done by different individuals, with different tumor types, different protocols... but all coming to a similar conclusion that does not support the somatic mutation theory. But the data more strongly support Otto Warburg's theory of disturbed energy metabolism.

So let's just look at a couple of these experiments. And, you know, the important point about this paper is: Don't let anyone tell you what they think about it. You're smart people! I tell people "Read the original paper and you come to your own conclusion. You make your own decision." Don't ask "Hey, what do you think of that paper? Do you like it or not? Yeah, maybe it's no good".

You can't believe how many people take in information second, third hand, rather than going to the original source. Read it! You make your decision if you like it! Do what Dr. Glassman did, hit me with a thousand questions and I'll be happy to answer them!

So let's look at some of the data:

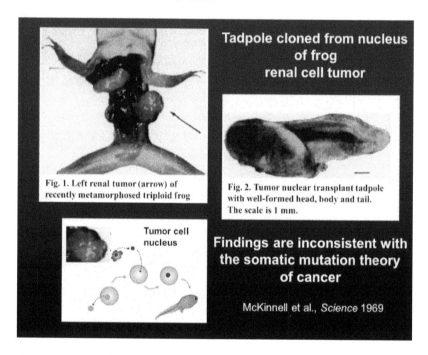

Tadpole cloned from nucleus of frog renal cell tumor

Fig. 1. Left renal tumor (arrow) of recently metamorphosed triploid frog

Fig. 2. Tumor nuclear transplant tadpole with well-formed head, body and tail. The scale is 1 mm.

Tumor cell nucleus

Findings are inconsistent with the somatic mutation theory of cancer

McKinnell et al., *Science* 1969

Now, this was done by McKinnell and his group, published in *Science* in 1969. I had the chance to speak with Dr. McKinnell before he passed away a couple years ago and we discussed these data at length.

So this frog has a massive renal tumor on the kidney. It's a kidney tumor, kills the frog, very aggressive. So what McKinnell and his group did is: They isolated cells from this kidney tumor and then they took the nucleus out of the kidney tumor cell and put it into a fertilized egg. The original nucleus of the egg was removed.

Here's the tumor cell, you take the nucleus that has the tumor suppressors and oncogenes and whatever - and you put it into this new cytoplasm that has normal mitochondria and you get a tadpole. And they looked very carefully, there was no evidence of the signature feature of cancer, dysregulated cell growth, anywhere. Everything looked perfectly normal.

10

The problem is, this tadpole could not fully develop into a mature frog. So whatever problem was in the tumor nucleus, it was not allowing the organism to fully mature. So the nuclear mutations didn't cause cancer, they blocked development.

These findings are inconsistent with the somatic mutation theory, which says, that the genes are causing the phenotype of dysregulated cell growth.

Another paper:

Reprogramming of a melanoma genome by nuclear transplantation

Konrad Hochedlinger,[1,4] Robert Blelloch,[1,2,4] Cameron Brennan,[3] Yasuhiro Yamada,[1] Minjung Kim,[3] Lynda Chin,[3,5] and Rudolf Jaenisch[1,6]

[1]Whitehead Institute for Biomedical Research, and Department of Biology, Massachusetts Institute of Technology, Cambridge, Massachusetts 02142, USA, [2]Department of Pathology, Brigham and Women's Hospital, Boston, Massachusetts 02115, USA, [3]Department of Medical Oncology, Dana-Farber Cancer Institute, Department of Dermatology, Harvard Medical School, Boston, Massachusetts 02115, USA

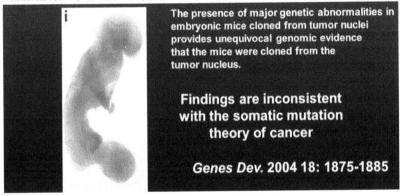

The presence of major genetic abnormalities in embryonic mice cloned from tumor nuclei provides unequivocal genomic evidence that the mice were cloned from the tumor nucleus.

Findings are inconsistent with the somatic mutation theory of cancer

Genes Dev. 2004 18: 1875-1885

I'm only going to give you information from a few of these studies, I put a whole bunch of these in the paper. It could take, you know, two days going over those experiments, but I'm just going to show you a few of them.

Now, this study was by Rudy Jaenisch and his colleagues at MIT. Rudy is one of the best and most preeminent developmental biologists. And he took these melanoma, malignant melanoma cells, and he characterized many of the mutations in the nucleus of the melanoma cell. They then he took the nucleus and made embryonic stem cells and cloned mice from the nucleus of melanomas.

He says here "The presence of major genetic abnormalities in embryonic mice cloned from the tumor nuclei provides unequivocal genomic evidence, that the mice were cloned from the tumor nucleus" - but they did not show any dysregulated cell growth. These findings are inconsistent with the somatic mutation theory of cancer.

And there was another series of experiments that were done by Dr. Wong and her group at Baylor College of Medicine, where they swapped the mitochondria from one cell to the next. These are much more difficult experiments than the nuclear transfer experiments.

So they take aggressive, malignant metastatic breast cancer cells, remove the mitochondria from the cytoplasm and bring in normal mitochondria from normal cells that don't have cancer. And the oncogenes and the abnormal growth was suppressed.

On the other hand, they took the mitochondria from the aggressive breast cancer cells and put them into an indolent cell (a type of low growth cancer) they exploded into high growth. So you've got a very different result. The mitochondria are calling the shots, not the nucleus!

So what we did to convey and summarize all of these data from all of these kinds of nuclear/mitochondrial transfer experiments in this simple diagram, which is now making its way through the web:

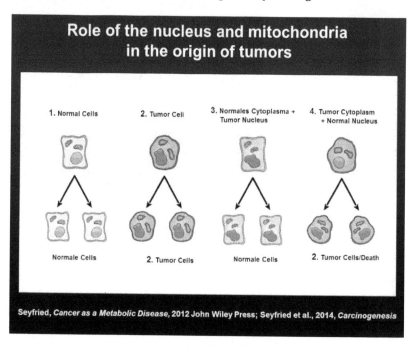

What I show here is: The green cell, which is a normal cell, begets normal cells. They have a normal genome, they have normal respiration. The red cell is the tumor cell. Tumor cells beget tumor cells. One tumor cell begets more tumor cells. They have genetic defects in the nucleus and they also have defects in the mitochondria.

Now, what is the origin of the disease? Is it the defects in the nucleus or is it the defects in the mitochondria? The nuclear transfer and mitochondrial transfer experiments provide evidence for this: Take the red nucleus and move it into the green cytoplasm - and you get normal cells that behave normally, grow normally, form normal tissues, sometimes organs and sometimes whole mice or frogs.

On the other hand Israel and Schaefer took the green nucleus and put it into the red cytoplasm. And in that case, you got either dead cells or tumor cells. You did not get normal cells. These are the exact opposite findings you would expect if the disease were a genetic disease!

Nuclear/mitochondrial transfer experiments are the strongest evidence to date that undermines the gene theory of cancer. The strongest evidence. No one has yet been able to explain how we get all these findings based on the somatic mutation theory of cancer!

So if that's the case: Why is the oncology field continuing to persist with therapies that are based on a flawed underlying hypothesis?

**If somatic mutations are not the origin of cancer,
how do we get cancer cells?**

Well, Otto Warburg described this a long time ago, back in the early part of the 20th century:

On the Origin of Cancer Cells
Otto Warburg (Science, 24 February, 1956)

Warburg Theory of Cancer

1. Cancer arises from damage to cellular respiration.

2. Energy through fermentation gradually compensates for insufficient respiration.

3. Cancer cells continue to ferment lactate in the presence of oxygen (Warburg effect).

4. Enhanced fermentation is the signature metabolic malady of all cancer cells.

- Cancer cells arise from damage to the respiration
- Energy through fermentation gradually compensates for the insufficient respiration
- Cancer cells continue to ferment lactic acid in the presence of oxygen

This is called the "Warburg Effect" and unfortunately the Warburg Effect has significantly confused this field, making it confusing to a lot of people. Because they said "Well, there's some tumor cells that don't show a Warburg Effect, therefore Otto Warburg must be wrong!"

Well, myself and some of my colleagues, we proposed that cancer cells can not only ferment sugar (glucose), but they can also ferment amino acids. And that amino acid is primarily glutamine, through the succinyl-CoA-ligase step and this is not well known to a lot of people. Basically, this is the missing link in Warburg's central theory.

So the cells are fermenting, but not only lactic acid, they can ferment amino acids and particularly glutamine. I'll present evidence for that.

- Enhanced fermentation is the signature metabolic malady of all cancer cells

Now, if we take a tumor and we look at this tumor and we separate the cells of the tumor: Every single cell in that tumor has a different genetic profile. No two cells in that tumor have the same kinds of mutations! This has been demonstrated over and over again.

However, every cell in that tumor is fermenting. Now, the question I ask to you: Is it more logical to focus on the common problem that exists in all of the cells of the tumor - or do you think it makes more sense to focus on the individual, unique differences of every cell in that tumor? Right? I mean, the answer should be clear.

But we do it wrong! We focus on the unique, individual differences at the expense of the common pathophysiology - and that's what we call the somatic mutation theory of cancer. Consequently, we get 1,600 people dying a day.

Now, let's look at this, energy:

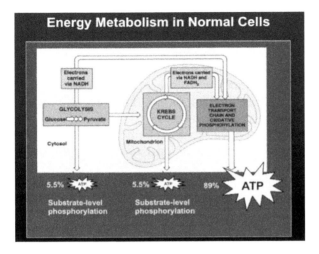

Alright. So, in a normal situation (this is a cartoon of just the mitochondria) most of the energy that we get in our body comes from breathing. About 89 to 90 percent through oxidative phosphorylation, respiration. We get smaller amounts of energy through these ancient pathways of substrate-level phosphorylation. In the cytoplasm, in the form of glycolysis and in the mitochondrial Krebs cycle through the succinyl-CoA-ligase step.

And we all know this, this is biochemistry, right? We're all breathing! We all are... well, I think. Any zombies out here? They don't breathe. But the issue is: Most of us breathe and when you exercise you breathe more and this is where we get our energy from, right?

Okay, now look at the cancer cell:

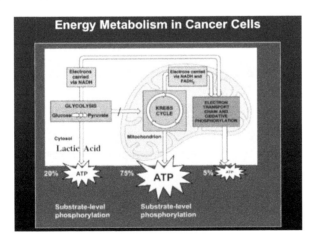

This is the same picture, but you'll notice that there's a major shift in where the energy is coming from. Much less energy is coming out of oxidative phosphorylation and a lot more is coming from these ancient, primitive pathways: substrate level phosphorylation.

And you see that... we now know, and we're learning more, that the majority of the energy is coming out of the mitochondria, but not through OxPhos [oxidative phosphorylation], but through the Krebs cycle. This is the new understanding that we're talking about, this is the missing link in Warburg's theory.

So tumors get a lot of energy from fermentation metabolism. Tumors can get energy without oxygen and this is where the cancer cells are getting their energy from! So people say "How do we get cancer then?" Well, all we have to do is take all of the data that was published in the cancer field over the last, you know, 100 years and just reconfigure it, along with Hanahan and Weinberg's *Hallmarks* paper.

Then we take the information and just rearrange the picture. And now we can put together, in a more logical way, the origin of "How we get cancer" - and once we know that, then we'll know how to manage the disease. It becomes much more clear to do that:

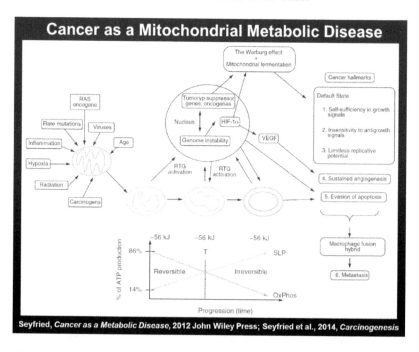

Seyfried, *Cancer as a Metabolic Disease*, 2012 John Wiley Press; Seyfried et al., 2014, *Carcinogenesis*

So what we have here on the on the left is the mitochondrion and people say "How do you get cancer?" Well, you can get cancer from any number of different things, right? Carcinogens cause cancer. You can get cancer if you're exposed to carcinogens. Radiation will cause cancer. Hypoxia (absence of oxygen) can cause cancer. Systemic inflammation, we heard that from Axel, he was telling us about the systemic inflammation and others.

Rare inherited mutations: People say "It must be genetic, because you got BRCA1 and P53... Angelina Jolie had her breasts and ovaries removed because of the BRCA1, she's trying to reduce her risk...

That's all secondary. It's secondary, because those BRCA1-mutations do not cause cancer, unless it damages the respiration. And there are people around that have BRCA1s who'll never get cancer, because the gene is not damaging the respiration.

Ras oncogene damages respiration.

Hepatitis C, and papilloma viruses enter mitochondria and damage the respiration. Age increases risk for cancer... so all these disparate risks factors was referred to as the oncogenic paradox, right?

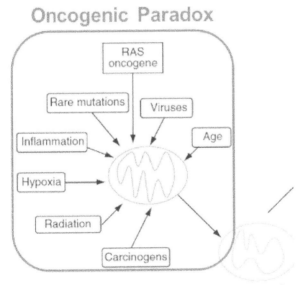

This was first pointed out by Albert Szent-Györgyi, who said "Hey, there's so many different ways to get cancer - but the common pathophysiological mechanism is not clear!" Well, once you understand that it's a mitochondrial metabolic disease, the mechanism becomes very clear!

And if you read Sid Mukherjee's book on the *Emperor of all maladies*, the one that was on the New York Times bestseller list, and it was the Pulitzer Prize-winning book on cancer... he struggles with this! If you read pages 285 and 303 in his book, he says "You know, it's just like, we don't... we just can't figure out how you get cancer from all these different things!"

You get cancer from all these different things, because they damage respiration and they form reactive oxygen species [ROS]. And reactive oxygen species are carcinogenic and mutagenic!

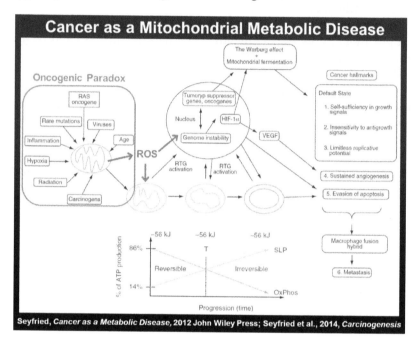

Seyfried, *Cancer as a Metabolic Disease*, 2012 John Wiley Press; Seyfried et al., 2014, *Carcinogenesis*

So the mutations that you see in the nucleus, that everybody is following - these red herrings - are all coming as a secondary cause to the damage to the respiration.

They are not the cause, they are the effects!

Alright? And then when the ROS are generated, they damage further the respiration, the cells are suffocating! Where are they going to get their energy? They have to upregulate substrate level phosphorylation.

So you see here at the bottom, the green line going down and the red line going up, substrate level phosphorylation. Which means a fermentation metabolism. So what are they fermenting? They're fermenting glucose and glutamine! Those are the two fuels that are driving up the energy. Because without energy nothing lives! Period!

Energy is everything. Without energy, you don't survive!

So what's happening with these cells is: They're shifting their energy away from respiration to a fermentation metabolism, using available fermentable fuels. So now we can put together all of the hallmarks of cancer in a more logical way, all linked back to damage to the respiration.

The first three hallmarks of Hanahan and Weinberg are all the result of the cell falling back on its default state, the state that the cells had before oxygen came into the atmosphere, some 2.5 billion years ago! Where everything on the planet was fermenting. They were fermenting amino acids and whatever else they can get!

And during that period of time the cells were in a state of unbridled proliferation and they would proliferate like crazy, until the fermentable fuels in the micro environment disappeared and they croaked. And they'd throw out all this waste material into the micro environment. In cancer this leads to vascularization or angiogenesis - another multi-billion dollar industry that's all based on, you know, indirect findings.

Okay. Then you say "Well, if this cancer cell is starting to suffocate, it should die, right?" Yeah, it should undergo programmed cell death and drop dead, that's called apoptosis. Why are they not undergoing apoptosis? Because the mitochondria control the apoptotic signaling system in the cell. Mitochondria are the cell's 'kill switch'! And your kill switch is broken and these cells are now bypassing apoptosis. They're not dying, they're proliferating.

So the big dog in this whole thing is metastasis. Okay, you know, I can agree with this. Where do you get metastasis from? Which is ultimately the biggest challenge in managing cancers, trying to control when it spreads through your body.

Now, you have to understand the biology of the disease. Once you understand the biology of the disease, you can start putting the pieces of the puzzle together:

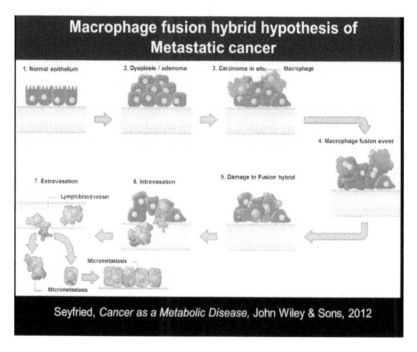

Seyfried, *Cancer as a Metabolic Disease*, John Wiley & Sons, 2012

Here's some blue cells, they're columnar epithelial cells. They could be in the breast, the colon or whatever. They get damaged by anyone of the provocative agents in the micro environment. They start entering the default state, they start proliferating.

Our body has a sensory system to know what's going on, this looks like an unhealed wound. So we have cells in our immune system that come into these places to heal wounds. And these are mostly macrophages. So they sense this, chemically, in the blood. They come in, out of the bloodstream, and they go right to these incipient cancer cells, growths of cells, to put out the fire, to heal the wound and then heal the tissue.

The problem is they throw out growth factors and cytokines, which are actually stimulatory towards these cells, which lost their growth control because of their fermentation behavior.

Now, they're making the situation worse, because it's the wrong context. What these red cells, our immune cells, do is to facilitate wound healing. They fuse together – they are very fusogenic cells, which is well documented in the scientific literature. So what's happening then with this continual fusion in this inflamed micro environment, is: You're diluting the cytoplasm of the red cell with the cytoplasm of the tumor cell, thereby shifting the immune cells from a respiratory system to a fermentation system, locked in.

These immune cells are already genetically programmed to enter and exit the bloodstream. You don't have to have this epithelial–mesenchymal transition, it makes absolutely no sense. (This is the gene theory explanation for metastasis.) This is the real thing! And we have evidence to support that in a number of different ways.

So you now have a rogue cell, part of our immune system, that's already programmed to spread through your body. Very difficult, they're already programmed to live in hypoxic environments, therefore anti-angiogenic drugs probably won't work - and they haven't worked.

So we now know the biology of the metastatic cell: It's a rogue macrophage! What do they eat? They eat glucose and glutamine! Okay. We know that.

Now, if most cancer cells obtain energy through fermentation, what therapies might be effective in managing tumors?

Well, one of the things, logically, is simply take away fermentable fuels and replace them in the body with non-fermentable fuels. And one of the ways to do that is: Stop eating! Calorie restriction [CR], ketogenic diets [KD], these kinds of things!

Calorie Restriction (CR) and Ketogenic Diets: A Metabolic Cancer Intervention

- CR involves a total dietary restriction

- CR differs from starvation

- CR maintains minerals and nutrients

- CR & KD reduce blood glucose and elevate ketone bodies, a non-fermentable fuel.

- CR & KD enhance mitochondrial biogenesis & OxPhos

- CR in mice equates to water-only fasting in humans

What calorie restriction and ketogenic diets do is:

- they differ from starvation
- they maintain normal levels of minerals
- they enhance mitochondrial biogenesis, and also, they replace fermentable fuels

You can't ferment ketone bodies! You need good respiration to obtain energy from ketone bodies. So you're going to remove or lower the glucose levels, and raise the ketone bodies which the normal cells are going to shift over to and the tumor cells are going to be marginalized because they can't use the ketone bodies!

And don't forget: We just heard from Michael about the basal metabolic rate. I do this in the mice. The mice, we give them 40% calorie restriction [CR] - but that's like water only fasting in humans, okay? People have to have to realize that because of the 7-fold difference in basal metabolic rate between mouse and human.

So ketogenic diets:

Composition (%) of the standard diet (SD) and the ketogenic diet (KD)

Components	Standard Diet (SD)	Ketogenic Diet (KD)
Carbohydrate	62	3
Fat	6	72
Protein	27	15
Energy (Kcal/gr)	4,4	7,2
F/ (P + C)	0,07	4

* The ketogenic diet should always be consumed in restricted amounts!

A lot of misinformation, a lot of misunderstanding. Basically, these are low-carb diets, high-fat diets. But it's the types of fats and proteins that play an important role.

Basically, you eat these diets in a restricted amount. The ketogenic diet, unfortunately it was labeled with the word 'diet', right? Whenever you put 'diet' on something, everything becomes like mysterious. It's a medicine! The ketogenic diet is a medicine, it's called *ketogenic metabolic therapy* and it should be respected as a medicine! If it's not used properly, it won't work, just like any medicine.

Not to say that it will harm you, but if you do eat too much ketogenic diet, you can in fact get insulin insensitivity. We worked in the epilepsy field for years and we understand how some of these diets can be not as effective as they should be.

But the whole strategy is not complicated, right? If the tumor cell needs fermentable fuel, then you take the fermentable fuel away from the tumor cell and you transition the body to a non-fermentable status:

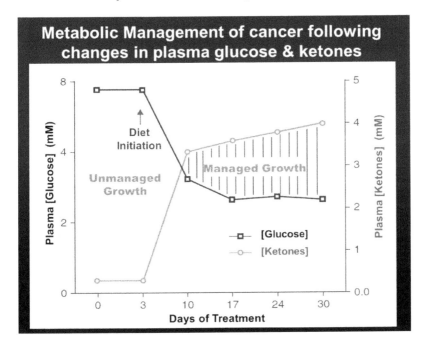

So you lower the blood sugar that the tumor cells need and you elevate ketone bodies, which the tumor cells can't use - but the normal cells can. You just simply marginalize the tumor.

Now, the tumor needs fuel, it can't live without energy. Where is it getting its fuel? It's fermenting. You're taking away a prime fuel - what's going to happen to those tumor cells? They're either going to die or they're going to slow down. And that's what happens!

Now, the first person that did this work was Linda Nebling, in a human situation, I should say:

Effects of a Ketogenic Diet on Tumor Metabolism and Nutritional Status in Pediatric Oncology Patients: Two Case Reports

Linda C. Nebling, PhD, MPH, RD, Flora Miraldi, MD, PhD, Susan B. Shurin, MD, and Edith Lerner, PhD, LD, FACN

Journal of the American College of Nutrition, Vol. 14, No. 2, 202–208 (1995)

The results showed that a ketogenic diet, which reduced blood glucose and elevated blood ketones, could provide long-term management in two children with recurrent inoperable brain tumors.

She took two little children, hopeless cases. Brutalized. Brutalized by the system. If you read her PhD dissertation, you'd be crushed about what they did to these little kids. They surgically mutilated them, gave them massive doses of chemo, radiation, all kinds of stuff. And they gave them up for hopeless, they said these kids aren't going to live more than two or three months.

She says "Can I try a ketogenic diet?" She was in nursing, getting her PhD in nursing. "Yeah, it's not going to do anything, they don't have long to live". So anyway, she rescued both of these kids! Their quality of life improved dramatically, they lived far longer than what was predicted. And it was based on the whole shift of the body's metabolism and I said "Wow, this is unbelievable!"

This was back in 1995 and I said to my students "You know, we should try some of that with our brain cancer and the mice!" And we were building these animal models, beautiful animal models of human brain cancers and we had the CT-2A, a neural stem cell tumor. Everybody's excited about neural stem cell cancers.

Anyway, we just gave them a standard diet [SD] - which is a high carb diet - but calorie restricted by 40%. Which is like a water-only therapeutic fast in humans:

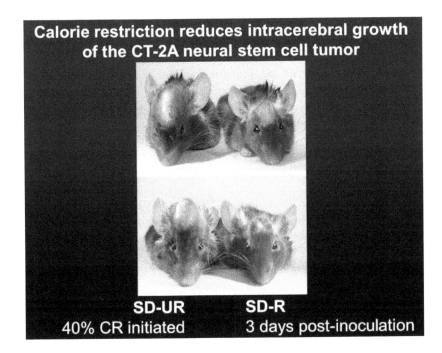

Calorie restriction reduces intracerebral growth of the CT-2A neural stem cell tumor

SD-UR   SD-R
40% CR initiated   3 days post-inoculation

And these tumors started to shrink big time! You know, go down 60 to 85 percent reduction in size.

And we said "Geez, what? Wow!" You know, I never saw anything like this before, so powerful, "What's going on?"

So then we analyzed, using linear regression analysis, using glucose as the independent variable, and either ketones or tumor weight as the dependent variables and glucose as the independent:

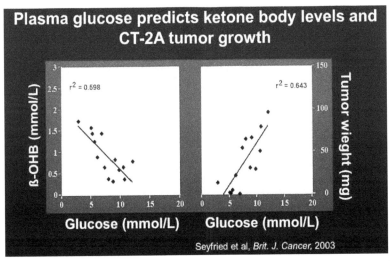

Plasma glucose predicts ketone body levels and CT-2A tumor growth

$r^2 = 0.598$

$r^2 = 0.643$

ß-OHB (mmol/L) — Glucose (mmol/L)

Tumor wieght (mg) — Glucose (mmol/L)

Seyfried et al, *Brit. J. Cancer*, 2003

Each square is an animal on a different diet. And you can see on the left here: As blood sugar goes down, ketones go up. And this is an evolutionarily conserved adaptation to food restriction. When our bodies are not getting the carbs, we're going to start mobilizing fats, bring them to the liver, chop them up, make water-soluble ketone bodies and these are going to go to the the tissues.

And on the right side: The blood sugar goes down, the size of the tumor goes down. The higher the sugar, the faster the tumor grows - the lower the glucose, the slower the tumor grows! Right?

So the higher the sugar, the faster your tumor grows.
The lower the sugar, the slower your tumor grows.

So if you want your tumor to grow fast, get your blood sugar up as high as it can get! Right? You go to oncology clinics and you see everybody eating ice cream and cake and candies! Don't they read the literature? This has been supported now in human gliomas, breast cancer, colon cancer... if you want your tumor to grow fast, get the sugar as high as it can go!

Now people say "Well, this looks wonderful and great, but we don't understand the mechanism." Bullshit! You understand the mechanism! We published so many papers and so many other people published papers on the mechanisms by which this works!

Calorie Restriction & KD Target Major Cancer Hallmarks

1. **Anti-angiogenic**
   Mukherjee et al., Clin. Cancer Res., 2004

2. **Anti-inflammatory**
   Mulrooney et al., PLOS One, 2011

3. **Pro-apoptotic**
   Mukherjee et al., Brit. J. Cancer 2002

It's anti-angiogenic, anti-inflammatory, pro-apoptotic. No cancer drug is known that can do this without toxicity! And therapeutic fasting can do it! So we and others have shown in many papers the molecular mechanisms by which this process works.

When you hear people say "Well, it's not proven!" – Well, they don't read the literature, nor do they contribute to it!

So this woman had this dog with a big mast tumor on his nose, right? Minka. You know, she listens to our YouTube videos and reads our regular papers. She's a lay person, doesn't have any training in medicine or anything.

This dog has this big tumor, she goes to the vet, who said "Well, yeah we're going to have to cut it out and then we're going to give radiation and chemo. 'about ten thousand dollars, maybe the dog will live seven more months. But it's going to be sick..." and blah blah, you know. The same stuff.

She said no. So she went to the butcher and she got the fresh chicken meat with the bones in it. Cut the calories by 40 percent, threw in some medium chain triglyceride [MCT] oil and some raw eggs in the mix. The dog lost about five percent of its body weight.

And you can see: The tumor started to shrink and disappear!

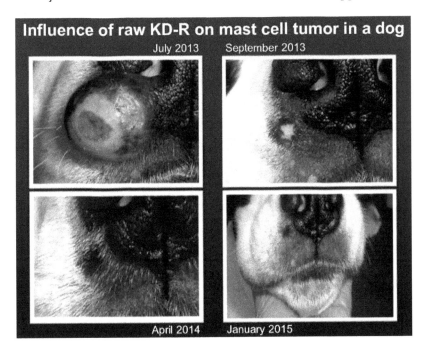

Influence of raw KD-R on mast cell tumor in a dog
July 2013 September 2013
April 2014 January 2015

And, you know, Minka is still alive today, doing fine! This was back in 2013. Impressive, how fast the dog responded, and there's many dogs now. They're putting them through these metabolic therapies that are doing really well.

Of course, the veterinarians were all over me about this. They don't think they should feed the raw meat to the dogs because of salmonella poisoning! Give me a break! I mean... have you ever seen what dogs eat? It's like, give me a break, you know! Salmonella poisoning!

So you're looking at this stuff and you're saying "Jesus!"... and then we did a YouTube video on this, about the dog cancer thing, got 5.3 million hits! Can you believe this? So there were all kinds of trolls out there, writing all these negative reports, giving me all kinds of grief. The hell with them, you know.

Okay. Now I want to talk about a really serious issue here, glioblastoma multiforme. And this is a really bad tumor with poor prognosis:

Glioblastoma Multiforme

- Among the most aggressive of all primary brain tumors

- Poor prognosis

- No effective therapies

- Composed of multiple cell types:
  Neoplastic Stem cells
  Neoplastic mesenchymal migroglia

- Highly Invasive, „Secondary Structures of Scherer"

- Metastatic outside the CNS

And unfortunately Senator John McCain is now struggling with this kind of a tumor. It's a nasty cancer, many multiple different kinds of cells, no effective therapy. So you get a whole bunch of different kinds of cells. Consequently the name "multiforme": Highly invasive.

So when you look at a brain tumor... here's a poor soul that sacrificed their brain for the study. And you can see: This nasty necrotic area, a cyst, large cyst:

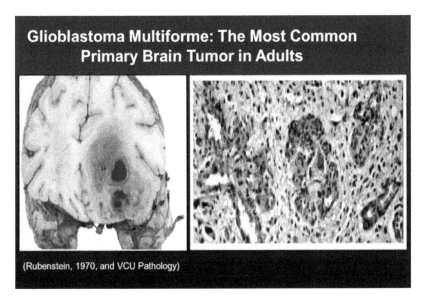

Glioblastoma Multiforme: The Most Common Primary Brain Tumor in Adults

(Rubenstein, 1970, and VCU Pathology)

But, if you look at the midline of the brain, you can see it shifted to the left. This is called "midline shift", okay?

So these tumors grow and they cause intercranial pressure. And people die from intracranial pressure, most of the people who have these kinds of tumors. The problem is: You can't surgically resect them, because the tumor cells have already spread out into the normal appearing brain areas. And the tumor cells use blood vessels as one of the mechanisms to disseminate: They go across the surface of blood vessels in the Virchow-Robin space.

So they use these blood vessels as kind of a railroad system to get through the brain. So it's very, very hard to do any kind of surgical resection. And you can see them, the dark blue cells around the blood vessels are the way... you can see on histology. Histology will tell you. This is how they spread through the brain and make it very difficult to get resolution.

And we all know that mitochondria are abnormal in brain cancer.

This picture shows an electron micrograph... the only way you can see mitochondria clearly is EM, electron microscopy:

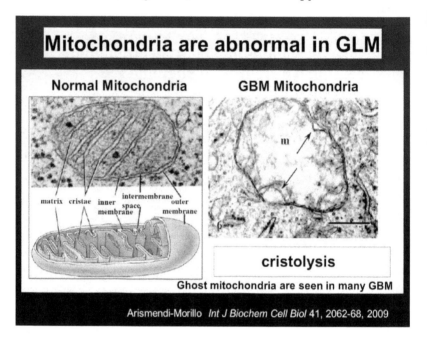

And the stripes in the mitochondria contain the proteins and the lipids of the electron transport chain, that allow us to get energy through oxidative phosphorylation. So you can see the nice stripes on the normal mitochondria there on the left. And the cristae are missing in GBM mitochondria, This is called cristolysis. The structure... the very structure of the organelle needed for oxidative phosphorylation is missing!!

Anybody can see the emptiness in that mitochondria. The stripes are missing! The stripes are missing, therefore the oxidative phosphorylation is missing, therefore the cell must ferment in order to survive. Everybody see that? Okay. There's a lot of papers in the literature showing that - yet, many members of my field say "The Mitochondria are normal". They obviously don't look at this or they don't want to see it.

The tumor cells ferment! They have to ferment, they don't have the structure. Structure dictates function. Without the structure, you can't get the function. The function is abnormal, because the structure is abnormal and my colleague Gabriel Arismendi-Morillo has published many beautiful papers on this.

So, if you can't get energy from oxidative phosphorylation, where do you get the energy to drive the beast? Where is that energy coming from? It's coming from glucose and glutamine - the two prime fuels that are going to drive the beast! They can't eat anything else! It's not there in sufficient quantity, we did the logistics on this.

These two fuels are abundant in the micro environment. So they come in, right? The two fuels together are synergistic:

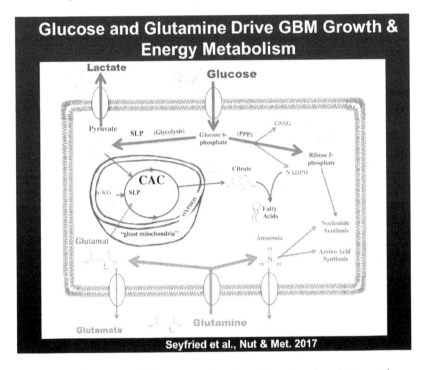

Glucose, glutamine. They come in, they fire the glycolytic pathway, the pentose pathway, the glutaminolysis pathway, deriving energy from substrate level phosphorylation. Making all of the stuff, the DNA-RNA proliferation... these cells grow like crazy.

So, what do we do in the clinic? Okay, so some poor soul comes in, diagnosed with a glioblastoma, devastating, you know. People don't know what they're going to do, you're just devastated. The patient's devastated, the family is devastated.

It's "My god, what's going on here?" - "Well, we have to do surgery, cut that tumor out right away!"

Sometimes you have to do that, when there's a herniation problem. But many times, you don't! You have a watchful waiting period. "No, no, no, we get them in as quickly as possible. We're going to debulk the tumor."

Surgeon takes out the tumor. Patient's sitting there, wakes up, "Oh, wow."

"Hey, how do you feel?"

"I feel pretty good."

"Okay. Now, as soon as you've recovered we're going to start giving you radiation therapy!"

So in the brain neurons and glia have a very close connection with each other. Intimate relationship, right? It's called the glutamine-glutamate cycle. It keeps our neurotransmitters in balance and everything is under control.

You break that glutamine-glutamate cycle, this happens:

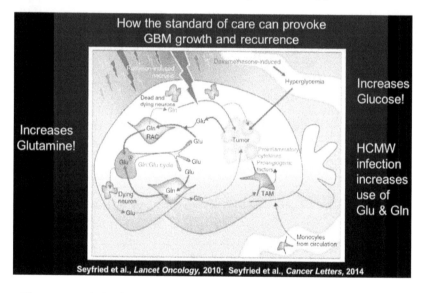

Seyfried et al., *Lancet Oncology*, 2010; Seyfried et al., *Cancer Letters*, 2014

Glutamate (which is an excitatory neurotransmitter) comes out, excites neurons, they die, you get necrotic death. Astrocytes take up the glutamate, turn it into glutamine.

Now, those tumor cells that have not been debulked will now sucking down the glutamine, created by not only the wound from the surgeon, but also by the radiation that's blowing the hell out of the micro environment in this tumor. Creating a vast amount of glutamine, which is one of the powerful fuels driving the beast, as I just said!

Now, when you take somebody and surgically resect the bulk of the tumor and then start radiating their brain, you start to get head swelling, brain swelling, from the radiation. Causing the heat, the edema. To reduce the edema we give them high dose steroids. High dose steroids create hyperglycemia! Right? Glucose! Glucose and glutamine are now created by the very procedures that are used to treat the patient!

To make matters worse, 90 percent of the brain tumor cells are infected with human cytomegalovirus, which is a supercharger for allowing the tumor cells to use glucose and glutamine!

I published this paper in *Lancet Oncology,* saying that the standard of care contributes to the growth and the recurrence of the tumor! Based on hard biochemical evidence! What do you think the response was? They don't want to hear about it!

Now, let's test the hypothesis about what I just said, okay?

Look at the results from treating patients with brain tumors with the standard of care:

GBM Patient Survival under current „Standard of Care"

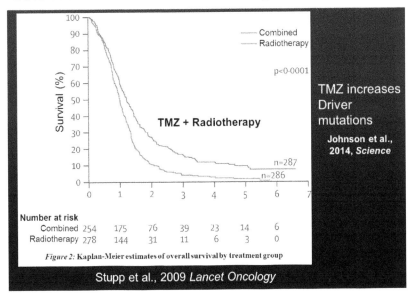

Figure 2: Kaplan-Meier estimates of overall survival by treatment group

Stupp et al., 2009 *Lancet Oncology*

So we have two lines here: The red line are those individuals that got radiation alone - and the blue line of those individuals who got radiation coupled with the toxic alkylating agent called Temozolomide [TMZ]. The fact that Temozolomide could contribute a little bit to survival was the single greatest advance in glioblastoma management in the last 50 years! Can you believe this? I was there, when they said this.

Now, look at the red line, the bottom line: The guys that got the radiation alone. How many survivors came out of the study? What's that number down at the end there? Zero! This has been reproduced.

You want to know about replicating data? This has been reproduced in every country in the world, over and over again. Nothing is more certain than irradiating people and having them all dead!

Now we throw in TMZ. "But hey, listen! TMZ is doing something!" Well, you get a few extra survivors from this. So, I said to myself and my students "What does TMZ do?" So we looked and we found out, the adverse effects of temozolomide are: Diarrhea, vomiting, nausea and fatigue. Wow! These are all indirect forms of calorie restriction!

So, we published and we said that we think that blip in survival rate is due to indirect calorie restriction. Do you think anybody ran out to test that hypothesis? No!

You know, Temozolomide also increases driver mutations. What the hell does that mean? Shouldn't Temozolomide make the tumors grow faster, if they increase driver mutations? We don't see that.

Now, let's put a face on this:

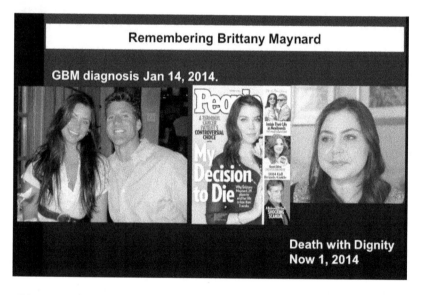

Okay, so this is Brittany Maynard. She was a young California girl, northern California, diagnosed with brain cancer in January 2014. The tumor was a small, a low-grade tumor. And within one month after taking out the low-grade tumor, it morphed into a glioblastoma multiforme.

She was then treated with "standard of care", heavy doses of steroids. And you can see her face on the right there, it looks totally different than when she just got married over here on the left. That's called "moonface", from overdosing steroids.

So she says "I'm out of here!" She's going to go to Oregon, next state up, and die with dignity with her family. She's going to throw the towel in!

And she put an article out, in *People Magazine* about her decision to die! The *People Magazine* article was all about the morality of death with dignity... nothing about the miserable failure of the standard of care that put her in that position in the first place!!

Now, what does it say when your patients kill themselves, rather than continue with your therapy? Not good!

Let's look at another face:

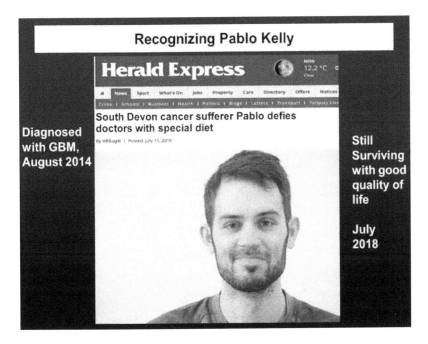

This is Pablo Kelly. Same age as Brittany, about 28. He was diagnosed with glioblastoma in August 2014. He emailed me and says "Can you help me? I don't want to take drugs, I don't want surgery, I don't want radiation. I don't want chemo!"

So, I gave him the kit that I send to most of the cancer patients who contact me. And I said "Hey, you might as well try it, Pablo!" - because he's like "I'm definitely not doing this stuff the doctors tell me!" He's from Devon, England.

He said "Okay, I'll try it your way!" So I gave him the kit. I hadn't heard from him, maybe a year and a half go by. All of a sudden, I get a letter from Pablo: "Oh geez, Pablo! Pablo is still alive!" And he had this big Youtube video, telling everybody how he was going to do keto and all this stuff. But anyway, he says, his now formerly inoperable tumor now has become operable.

So he asked me about it and I said, "Well, if you can shrink it down, get it out Pablo!" So he goes and has the surgery. It was earlier this year, he gets the tumor out. He's had few seizures, but his quality of life is pretty good. His wife just had a baby. He's still alive, he's doing well. Right?

He has a quality of life, he's alive!

So what we did, knowing about all these situations: We built the 'Glucose Ketone Index Calculator' [GKI]. Which helps patients and others get into therapeutic ketosis. So if you want to stop the growth of the tumor, the first step you got to do is:

Get into therapeutic ketosis!

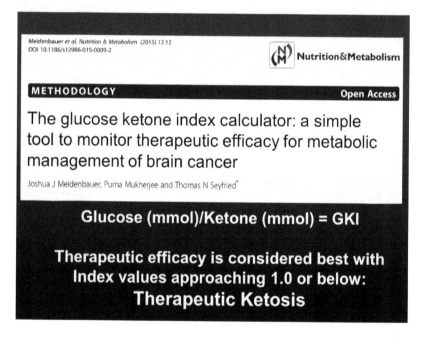

Meidenbauer *et al. Nutrition & Metabolism* (2015) 12:12
DOI 10.1186/s12986-015-0009-2

(N)(M) Nutrition&Metabolism

METHODOLOGY   Open Access

The glucose ketone index calculator: a simple tool to monitor therapeutic efficacy for metabolic management of brain cancer

Joshua J Meidenbauer, Purna Mukherjee and Thomas N Seyfried*

Glucose (mmol)/Ketone (mmol) = GKI

Therapeutic efficacy is considered best with Index values approaching 1.0 or below: Therapeutic Ketosis

And it's the ratio of glucose millimolar / ketone millimolar, with one of these Precision Extra or Keto-Mojo meters. We're testing all these things against chemistry.

The GKI number helps patients stop the growth of the tumor! So it makes it easier, rather than trying to measure the two fuels together, you get a single value.

We also built some of the greatest preclinical glioma models... the most replicable models to human glioblastoma, spontaneous brain tumors in the mouse. So you know that they're coming from the host

And you can see this mouse, VM-M3 is a glioblastoma. On the left here you can see the tumor:

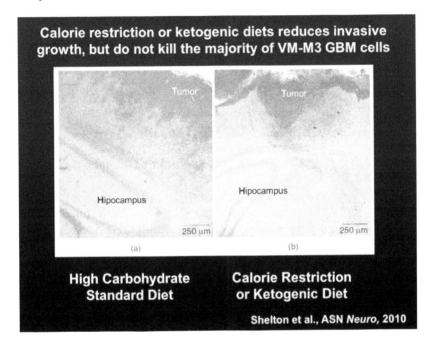

Calorie restriction or ketogenic diets reduces invasive growth, but do not kill the majority of VM-M3 GBM cells

Tumor

Tumor

Hipocampus

Hippocampus

250 μm

250 μm

(a)

(b)

High Carbohydrate Standard Diet

Calorie Restriction or Ketogenic Diet

Shelton et al., ASN *Neuro*, 2010

It invades right through the brain using the same mechanisms as you see in humans. On the right is the same tumor in mice, treated with calorie restriction and ketogenic diets. We pound these tumors, hard! Now, we stopped invasion. You can see on the right, there's much less invasive behavior - but we couldn't kill the cells. They're still growing!

I threw everything at these tumors, we were fasting these mice, we were bringing the sugars down, ketones up and the damn tumor cells are still alive! Humans do much better than these mice. I tell you, I don't understand how the human brain can respond so well. Humans are much more responsive to this therapy than the mice. People say "You cure mice all the time!" You don't cure these mice! A mouse that has the same tumor as a human, you get the same problem.

So, I said "These tumors must be using glutamine!" So, we tested the glutamine hypothesis by using 6-Diazo-5-oxo-L-norleucine which is DON. It's been used in the past, it's an old drug, it was used years ago. It worked out for some cancers but not for other cancers, you know. It was just one of those things... some were a little too toxic, some not toxic.

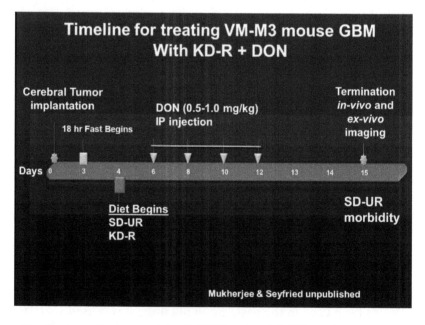

Anyway, what it does is: It stops glutamine metabolism! So we decided to test mice with DON.

We decided to put the tumors into the brain and then let it go for three days until the tumors are raging. Then put them on a fast and then switch them back either to a high carbohydrate [Standard Diet unrestricted calories SD-UR] diet or a ketogenic diet, restricted [KD-R], with or without DON:

On the top, then, we pulsed DON, pulsed DON at day 6, 8, 10, 12, every other day. We'd give them a little DON while they were on these

38

diets. We stopped the experiments at day 15 because the control mice, they're dying! They're starting to get morbid, because the tumors are growing so fast from all the carbohydrates and everything!

We then compare and contrast the brain tissues and the biochemistry of the tumors at 15 days. And I have to add... we genetically engineered these tumor cells to be bioluminescent so we can see how active the tumor is by putting them into a bioluminescence Xenogen machine. We take the brains out of the mice and we put them in these petri dishes and put some luciferin in there:

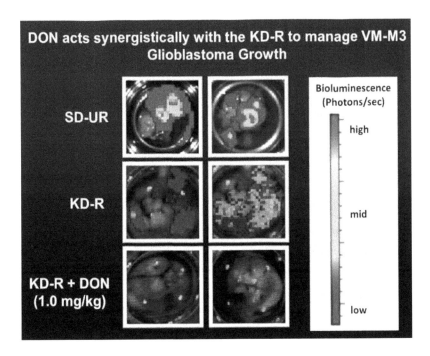

The light tells us how many living tumor cells there are in the brains of these mice that are treated under these different conditions. And the mice on the top: You see a lot of bright lights, reds and yellows and all this... They're the ones that didn't get anything but the high carb diet. They're tumors are raging! And we have a lot of different studies to show this.

The ketogenic diet, restricted: You can still see, there's a lot of living tumor cells in the brains of these mice! We did not cure these mice with ketogenic diets. The tumor cells did not invade as much, and I'll show you evidence for that.

But when you add the DON, the glutamine inhibitor, together with the diet we got no light! Right? There was no light! We did this over and over again!

Here's the data of a series of individual mice:

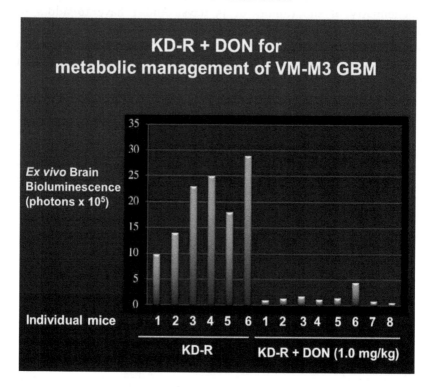

1-6 are the guys that got the diet only [KD-R] and then the other guys, 1-8, got the diet with the DON. And that background light at the +DON group, that's all background except for one mouse there with a little breakthrough light. But by and large, we really eliminated the light and the living cells in these tumors by putting the diet together with the DON!

The DON by itself is okay, but it doesn't get rid of as much light as as putting the DON with the diet. The two together work best. And of course, the gold standard for determining cancer is histology! That's what they, do they take needle biopsies "Oh, you look at the cells you got cancer", right? So you have to do histology to determine what's going on inside the tissue.

And when we did that... here we have the standard diet, the ketogenic diet restricted and the ketogenic diet restricted with the DON:

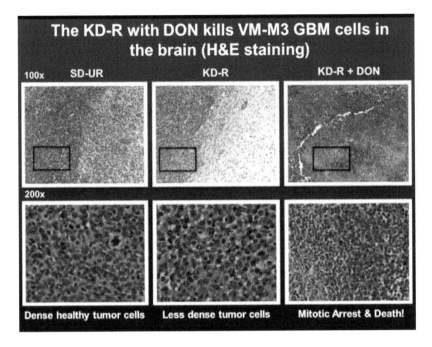

The KD-R with DON kills VM-M3 GBM cells in the brain (H&E staining)

100x   SD-UR   KD-R   KD-R + DON

200x

Dense healthy tumor cells   Less dense tumor cells   Mitotic Arrest & Death!

Low power, high power, is what you're seeing. And if you look at the standardized diet on the left, these cells are piled on top of each other. They can't grow any faster than they're growing! The mitotic figures, the cells are densely packed. And that's what you get when you have a high carbohydrate diet.

The ketogenic diet, the one in the middle, you can see the white part of the brain there: That's the normal part. And KD is blocking the invasion from the dark blue into the white. You can see how much the invasion is over here in the high carb diet. The cells are spaced further apart. So what it's telling us is: The KD is preventing invasion and it's stopping the rate of growth. But they're still growing.

On the far right, you've got the DON and... what we see is: All dead cells! Right? Blasted, the treatment slaughtered these cancer cells! They're all broken, mitotic arrest, they're all dead! This supports the fact that we didn't have any light, the tumor cells are dead!

So based on this we developed the "Press Pulse Therapeutic Strategy" for humans:

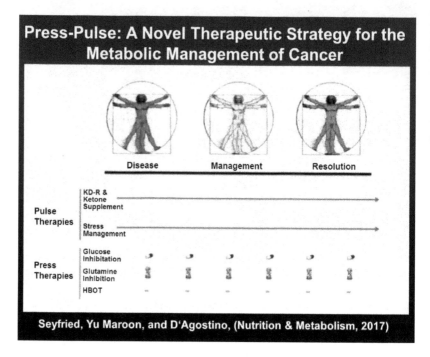

Press-Pulse: A Novel Therapeutic Strategy for the Metabolic Management of Cancer

Seyfried, Yu Maroon, and D'Agostino, (Nutrition & Metabolism, 2017)

Based on our pre-clinical studies in mice. And I worked together with Dom D'Agostino, Joe Maroon the neurosurgeon. George Yu is an oncologist. And we put this together and, unfortunately I don't have time to tell you where the origin of press-pulse comes.

But basically: We use press therapies, which can include the ketogenic diet, restricted, ketone supplementation - and stress management!

You know... you can't believe that when you have cancer people get stressed out! You have this impending doom,"I'm going to die!" What does that do? It raises your blood sugar - cortisol goes up! You've got to have stress management! So we use exercise, we use music therapy, we use yoga therapy. Whatever works to lower the stress of the individual.

We use the diet as a press: The diet is controlling the availability of sugar to the cancer - and raising ketones, that the tumor cells can't use. Once we get the patient into therapeutic ketosis and lowered stress, we then apply pulses. And we use drugs like 2-Deoxy-D-Glucose, insulin potentiation therapy... we then hit them with glutamine inhibitors, like EGCG (the green tea extract) and chloroquine (the anti-inflammatory). And we would like to get DON, of course, and other drugs.

Then we put them in hyperbaric oxygen chambers [HBOT]. Hyperbaric oxygen will kill tumor cells (just like radiation does) without toxicity! Once you have removed the glucose and glutamine, get the patient into therapeutic ketosis!

So, we can replace the entire standard of care with a logical therapeutic process, that's non-toxic. And we gradually move the patient from the disease state to the so-called "managed state". And eventually, hopefully, to a long-term management and possible resolution using press-pulse metabolic therapy.

Now, how does it work? Okay, so here's a paper that we just published on a patient with glioblastoma from Egypt. We can't do this in the United States!! You can't do this in England, right? You can't do it in a lot of places because of the obligatory standard of care protocol!

So, we had to go to Egypt, where they read our books, they read our stuff and they said "Okay, we're going to try this!" They came to me and told me how they're doing this and they said "Can you help us write it all up?" You know, a lot of physicians can't write papers. But I do this for a living.

I said "We'll get the data, we'll put it all together, just like we do the mice and we'll set up a protocol":

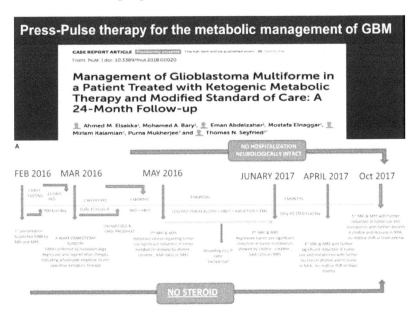

Management of glioblastoma to patients with ketogenic metabolic therapy with modified, modified standard of care. That's what we can't do in this country, so far: IRBs will not allow us to modify the standards of care.

We took this guy, he came in, his whole left side was dragging... he was a metabolic mess, he had pre-diabetes, he had low Vitamin D, had all kinds of other issues... besides, he had a glioblastoma.

So, the first thing Dr. Elsakka did: We gave him a 3 day water only fast and then transitioned the guy to a 900 kilocalorie a day ketogenic diet for 21 days. So he's out over 3 weeks, before we touched him!

Then he did a wake craniotomy. We debulked the tumor! The tumor looks different now! The tumor has a different morphology based on the on the treatment of the diet up front. You're shrinking down those cells!

Then, for another 3 months, we gave him chloroquine, we gave him ECGC, we gave hyperbaric oxygen... Then we were forced into doing standard of care. Because they have to do it! And while he's getting the standard of care - which is radiation and chemo - he's also on hyperbaric oxygen and the diet as well.

And then, for another three months, you can see after that... Now, at 24 months, the guy is doing fine, right? He's a corn farmer, he's back out working in the fields. So now he's out 30 months and he's still doing. I just talked to Dr. Elsakka the other day, I asked "How's the guy doing, the corn farmer?"

"He's doing fine!"

But he had a little radiation edema which pisses us all off some fierce. You don't want to irradiate the human brain, under any conditions! I don't understand that, it kills me! You know, I'm looking at these poor people and I'm saying

"What are you doing?"

"Well, we have to kill the tumor cells!"

"Just take away the glucose and glutamine you get the same effect!"

So here you can see the effect of our treatment:

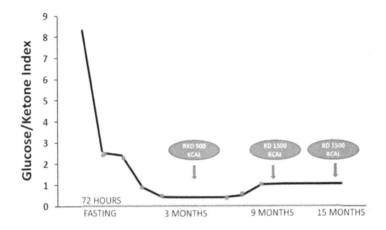

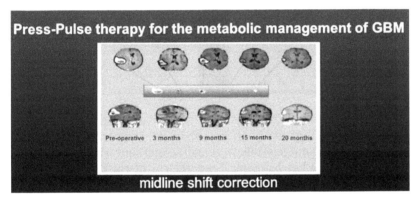

Bring the GKI down, glucose ketone index, we got it down really nice, therapeutic ketosis. And on the bottom, look at this: You see the red line on the bottom, see this big tumor there? Okay. Watch as the treatment continues at the very end, you see the red line in the middle is now straight! We corrected the midline shift and the guy's doing fine!

And it's just not brain cancer. This is a patient for a triple negative breast cancer from our colleagues in Turkey, in the Istanbul Clinic. And they're treating all kinds of lung cancer, pancreatic cancer... all stage four, all stage four cancers. This stage four woman comes in with a triple negative breast cancer:

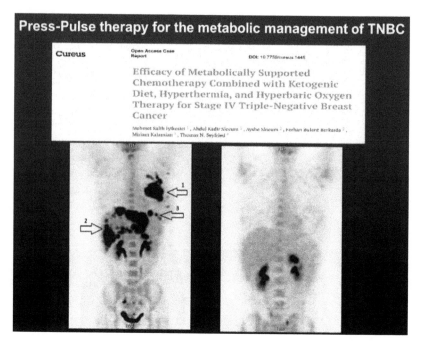

Press-Pulse therapy for the metabolic management of TNBC

Cureus   Open Access Case Report   DOI: 10.7759/cureus.1445

Efficacy of Metabolically Supported
Chemotherapy Combined with Ketogenic
Diet, Hyperthermia, and Hyperbaric Oxygen
Therapy for Stage IV Triple-Negative Breast
Cancer

Mehmet Salih Iyikesici [1], Abdul Kadir Slocum [2], Ayshe Slocum [2], Ferhan Bulent Berkarda [2], Miriam Kalamian [3], Thomas N. Seyfried [4]

Number one is in the breast, two is in the liver, three is in soft muscle tissue. Again, ketogenic diets, hypothermia, hypobaric oxygen... the lowest dose of chemo possible to remain compliant with the law! I said to Dr. Slocum "What happens if we get rid of the chemo?" "Patient would do better!" But you got to do it! Because you're going to lose your license if you don't. Can you believe this?

Anyway, this patient is doing well! We published in *Cureus Open Access*. We got asked by somebody "How's that patient doing, how's that patient?" Dr. Slocum says the patient is still doing well. Never lost hair, always had a high quality of life, never got sick. And we're seeing this over and over again.

Not in everybody! I don't want to make it look like "Hey, everybody's doing well!" You know, there's a few people who don't make it. They've been beat up so bad by the traditional standards of care, their bodies can't rally. They're so demolished in their ability to heal themselves by the traditional standards of care, they can't heal, they can't rally.

So we have this, GBM and other stage four cancers. I don't consider them as terminal cancers! I don't think they should be considered terminal cancers, okay? Because we're mistreating the patients. We're putting them into risk of death by the very treatments that we're using to try to save them. Makes no sense. You poison and irradiate people to make them healthy? Give me a break!

You've got Brittany Maynard "standard of care" - and then you got Pablo, rejects standard of care. "Oh. They're only one person."

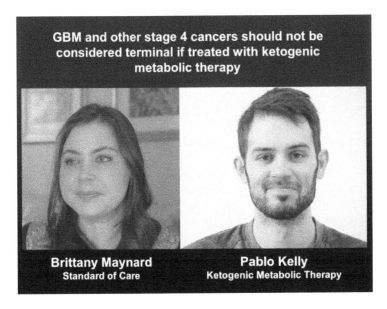

No, there's not one... there's Allison Gannett, there's Andrew Scarborough, there's a whole bunch out there - we just haven't published them yet!

So, Conclusions:

- Cancer is a type of mitochondrial metabolic disease. It's not a genetic disease!

Okay? This misunderstanding is the greatest tragedy in the history of medicine. Leading to the unnecessary suffering and death of tens of millions of people! By a fundamental misunderstanding of what the nature of the disease is!

- These cells rely on substrate level phosphorylation.

It's the hallmark of what these cells do!

- They're dependent on glucose and glutamine as the prime fuels for GBM and all these other cancers.

They need that fermentable fuel! **Who's targeting the fermentable fuels? Nobody!**

- The Press-Pulse metabolic therapy is non-toxic, cost-effective for the management and possible resolution of all types of cancers

It's a singular disease, all these tumor cells are all fermenters. Doesn't make any difference. It's my opinion and it could be, you know... I don't know if I'll live to see it.... that this strategy will eventually make all of the strategies obsolete. It's just a matter of time.

So I want to thank my collaborators and colleagues from the United States, from Turkey, from Germany, from Venezuela, from Hungary, Greece, France, Egypt, India and China. The Chinese want to now start dovetailing this into their traditional Chinese medicine.

And I especially like to thank our supporters and the funding that we get from them - which is very hard, believe me!

You get massive amounts of money to study cancer, you get very little if you want to try to resolve the disease!

Single Cure Single Cause Foundation [now *The Foundation for Metabolic Cancer Therapies*], CrossFit - thank you very much. Dr. Joe Maroon, team surgeon for the Pittsburgh Steelers, distinguished neurosurgeon at the University of Pittsburgh. George Yu, oncologist. Ellen Davis, Boston College. And in the past the NIH.

Thank you for your attention.

Dr. Thomas Seyfrieds book and paper:

Seyfried, *Cancer as a Metabolic Disease*, 2012 John Wiley Press;

_____

Cancer as a metabolic disease: implications for novel therapeutics

Thomas N. Seyfried,* Roberto E. Flores, Angela M. Poff and Dominic P. D'Agostino - *Carcinogenesis*. 2014 Mar

https://www.ncbi.nlm.nih.gov/pmc/articles/PMC3941741/

Papers cited / mentioned (in chronological order):

1. Hallmarks of cancer: the next generation
Douglas Hanahan, Robert A Weinberg
Cell. 2011 Mar 4
https://pubmed.ncbi.nlm.nih.gov/21376230/

2. A comprehensive catalogue of somatic mutations from a human cancer genome
Erin D. Pleasance, R. Keira Cheetham, Michael R. Stratton
Nature. 463
https://www.nature.com/articles/nature08658

3. Transplantation of pluripotential nuclei from triploid frog tumors
R. G. McKinnell, B. A. Deggins, D. D. Labat
Science. 1969 Jul 25
https://pubmed.ncbi.nlm.nih.gov/5815255/

4. Reprogramming of a melanoma genome by nuclear transplantation
Konrad Hochedlinger, Robert Blelloch, Cameron Brennan et al.,
Genes Dev. 2004 Aug 1
https://pubmed.ncbi.nlm.nih.gov/15289459/

5. On the Origin of Cancer Cells
Otto Warburg
Science. 24 Feb 1956
https://science.sciencemag.org/content/123/3191/309

6. Effects of a ketogenic diet on tumor metabolism and nutritional status in pediatric oncology patients: two case reports
L. C. Nebeling, F. Miraldi, S. B. Shurin, E. Lerner
J Am Coll Nutr. 1995 Apr 14
https://pubmed.ncbi.nlm.nih.gov/7790697/

7. Role of glucose and ketone bodies in the metabolic control of experimental brain cancer.
T. N. Seyfried , T. M. Sanderson, M. M. El-Abbadi, R. McGowan, P. Mukherjee
Br J Cancer. 2003 Oct 6
https://pubmed.ncbi.nlm.nih.gov/14520474/

8. Antiangiogenic and proapoptotic effects of dietary restriction on experimental mouse and human brain tumors

Purna Mukherjee , Laura E. Abate, Thomas N. Seyfried
Clin Cancer Res. 2004 Aug 15
https://pubmed.ncbi.nlm.nih.gov/15328205/

9. Influence of caloric restriction on constitutive expression of NF-κB in an experimental mouse astrocytoma
Tiernan J. Mulrooney, Jeremy Marsh, Ivan Urits, Thomas N. Seyfried, Purna Mukherjee
PLoS One. 2011 Mar 30
https://pubmed.ncbi.nlm.nih.gov/21479220/

10. Dietary restriction reduces angiogenesis and growth in an orthotopic mouse brain tumour model
P. Mukherjee, M. M. El-Abbadi, J. L. Kasperzyk, M. K. Ranes, T. N. Seyfried
Br J Cancer. 2002 May 20
https://pubmed.ncbi.nlm.nih.gov/12085212/

11. Electron microscopy morphology of the mitochondrial network in human cancer
Gabriel Arismendi-Morillo
Int J Biochem Cell Biol. 2009 Oct
https://pubmed.ncbi.nlm.nih.gov/19703662/

12. Does the existing standard of care increase glioblastoma energy metabolism?
Thomas N. Seyfried, Laura M. Shelton, Purna Mukherjee
Lancet Oncol. 2010 Sep 11
https://pubmed.ncbi.nlm.nih.gov/20634134/

13. Effects of radiotherapy with concomitant and adjuvant temozolomide versus radiotherapy alone on survival in glioblastoma in a randomised phase III study: 5-year analysis of the EORTC-NCIC trial
Stupp R et al.,
Lancet Oncol. 2009 May 10
https://pubmed.ncbi.nlm.nih.gov/19269895/

14. The glucose ketone index calculator: a simple tool to monitor therapeutic efficacy for metabolic management of brain cancer
Joshua J. Meidenbauer, Purna Mukherjee, Thomas N. Seyfried
Nutr Metab (Lond). 2015 Mar 11
https://pubmed.ncbi.nlm.nih.gov/25798181/

15. Calorie restriction as an anti-invasive therapy for malignant brain cancer in the VM mouse
Laura M. Shelton, Leanne C. Huysentruyt, Purna Mukherjee, Thomas N. Seyfried
ASN Neuro. 2010 Jul 23
https://pubmed.ncbi.nlm.nih.gov/20664705/

16. Therapeutic benefit of combining calorie-restricted ketogenic diet and glutamine targeting in late-stage experimental glioblastoma
Purna Mukherjee, Thomas N. Seyfried et al.,
Commun Biol. 2019 May 29
https://pubmed.ncbi.nlm.nih.gov/31149644/

17. Management of Glioblastoma Multiforme in a Patient Treated With Ketogenic Metabolic Therapy and Modified Standard of Care: A 24-Month Follow-Up
Ahmed M. A. Elsakka, Thomas N. Seyfried et al.,
Front Nutr. 2018; 5; 20
https://www.ncbi.nlm.nih.gov/pmc/articles/PMC5884883/

Chapter 2: Dr. Dominic D'Agostino on the ketogenic diet and the press-pulse treatment for cancer

(...)

These are the applications for the ketogenic diet and there are many applications that I didn't even put on here:

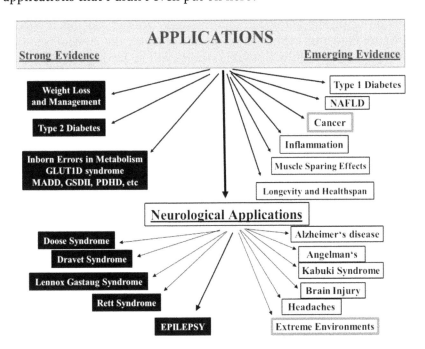

Like the ketogenic diet for acne or polycystic ovary syndrome [PCOS]. Or we study various psychological effects of ketones, too.

So I am just going to focus primarily on cancer... but just look at the emerging applications. And on the left here are things that have really strong evidence in the literature.

Weight loss and weight management, type 2 diabetes I think we can say there's strong evidence for that. Obviously inborn errors of metabolism. The last prior to coming here, I was in Chicago meeting with the doctors who actually give ketones intravenously with all these different neuro-metabolic disorders and they can bring children to life by giving them ketones when they have specific metabolic disorders.

And things like Lennox-Gaustaug syndrome, it's been used for decades for that disorder in epilepsy. I have it in the emerging applications but I think type 1 diabetes, too - there's emerging data from people out there using it. like the group "Typeonegrit" on Facebook.

My PhD student is part of that group and there was a publication that essentially resulted from that group. So there's more data emerging.

And in cancer: 10 years ago, I think there was one or two studies on ClinicalTrials.gov and now I looked this week, there's over 30 clinical trials on using the ketogenic diet in cancer studies. So this is a very emerging field and I think you're gonna see with the current clinical trials, a lot more results from this studies will be hitting PubMed.

It was observations that we made in the cell types that we studied under hyperbaric oxygen therapy and also with supplemental ketones... we observed that ketones decreased proliferation in these cancer cell types that led me down this path:

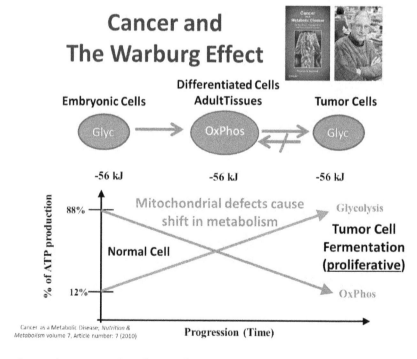

I wasn't supposed to be studying it, I was supposed to be studying oxygen toxicity seizures because we had a contract with the Navy and I was full-time on that contract. But I was obsessed with these observations that we made in cancer cells. And the only thing that really explained the observations that we saw was the Warburg Effect.

Especially the damaged mitochondria and the overproduction of oxygen free radicals as we increased oxygen concentration. And no one had seen that before because no one has a microscope inside a hyperbaric chamber, so these are some novel observations and I needed to explain them. And it connected me with several people including Dr. Tom Seyfried at Boston College.

I read his review shortly after connecting with him, *Cancer as a Metabolic Disease*, which he published in *Nutrition & Metabolism* and then he's got a book by the same name *Cancer as a Metabolic Disease*.

I have published at least seven articles or studies with Tom Seyfried, he explained to me the Warburg Effect which... I had taken cancer biology in college and I had never heard of it before! That cancer metabolism is fundamentally different from metabolism of healthy cells.

Essentially the Warburg Effect in one sentence is damaged mitochondrial respiration and there's compensatory fermentation. So the basic energy processes that allow a cell to maintain its bioenergetic potential would be oxidative phosphorylation. The mitochondria is making about 88 to 90% of the ATP, the energy currency in the cell. In neurons and heart and skeletal muscle, too.

And as a person or the cells are exposed to a number of different agents, they could be
- chemicals
- radiation
- inflammation
- hypoxia
- insulin resistance and
- hyperglycemia

these agents produce a very ripe ripe environment for the mitochondria to be damaged and the mitochondria-DNA to be damaged.

The nucleus has very robust DNA repair mechanisms. The mitochondria does not have as robust DNA repair mechanisms. So if a cell is bombarded with things like radiation or carcinogenic agents, the capacity for the mitochondria to repair itself is not as as high, is not as robust as the the nucleus's ability to repair DNA.

So the mitochondria take a big hit. And as mitochondrial function is impaired by progressive damage from environmental agents... viruses, for example, can cause cancer. And the viruses that cause cancer impair mitochondrial function!

So mitochondrial function goes down, cellular ATP levels go down and the nucleus of the cell can sense the bioenergetic potential of the cell, it can sense the ATP levels - and it senses that the cells is in an energetic crisis.

And when it gets to this threshold, I would say... and every cell is different, every person is different. I mean, there's a lot of variables here. But there comes a threshold where progressive damage to mitochondrial function causes a cascade of events to activate a number of genomic pathways that stimulate the cell to increase glycolysis. And various oncogenes are associated with increased glucose metabolism. So a normal cell then transforms and...

We also have to understand that embryonic cells that are proliferating and growing fast also have a glycolytic phenotype. But normal cells that are not proliferating primarily get their energy from mitochondrial oxidative phosphorylation. When the mitochondria are damaged by a number of different agents they will transform. I believe that hyperglycemia, hyperinsulinemia, mitochondrial syndrome is a major driver for this mitochondrial damage.

When the cell transitions from an oxidative phosphorylation energy pathway to a more glycolytic pathway through mitochondrial damage then there's a point of no return. It transitions from a normal cell to a tumor cell. It's debated, but it's not fully understood, if a tumor cell can transition back to a healthy cell. Generally, we don't believe that that can happen, maybe in some cases it can.

But when a normal cell is activated and an oncogenic program and drivers are kicked on, it becomes a tumor cell. And there are a number of factors that can drive the Warburg Effect and actually make that tumor an expanding biomass to a large solid tumor. And drivers of the Warburg Effect can kick on invasiveness and metastasis where those tumor cells get in the circulation and then metastasize. Then it becomes sort of an irreversible process.

So these are the drivers of the Warburg Effect and maybe, I guess Tom Seyfried would say the 'initiators' of the Warburg Effect:

Drivers of the Warburg Effect

- Damaged mitochondria
- Tumor hypoxia
- Elevated Insulin, glucose, lactate
- Increased PI3K/AKT/mTOR
- Elevated ROS and inflammation
- Suppressed anti-tumor immunity

The metabolic theory of cancer posits that it's the initial damage to the mitochondria that's the enabling factor that essentially transitions a normal cell to a cancer cell. There are genes involved, no doubt. But the metabolic control of those genes is likely the root cause.

And now, the geneticists... you know, in years passed it was just linked to genetic alterations. But now we have an appreciation and an understanding (and NIH directed research) to understand how metabolism is directing those gene pathways to actually initiate carcinogenesis and the factors associated with cancer progression, too.

So damaged mitochondria within the theory of metabolic theory of cancer is the initial cause and also a major driver. There's a derangement of tumor metabolism.

Tumor hypoxia: As a tumor expands, as the biomass expands, the core of that tumor becomes hypoxic, damages the mitochondria more, there's more genetic mutations and the inside of the tumor takes on a more aggressive Warburg phenotype. So it's literally fermenting sugar as it grows.

And really people with advanced tumors if they look at the actual tumor, the mitochondria are defficient, they are structurally and biochemically abnormal. And according to Dr. Seyfried and some of the colleagues that I've connected with, when it comes to aggressive tumors they have never found a tumor that has what we would call 'normal' mitochondria!

Damaged mitochondria are really a major driver of cancer. If your mitochondria are healthy they call the shots! Healthy mitochondria will keep a high bioenergetic state of the cell, high ATP levels will enhance the fidelity of the nuclear genome such that DNA repair processes will happen and preserve that genomic stability.

So that's a really important point I think that Tom Seyfried tries to make: The ultimate tumor suppressors are healthy mitochondria. There are different ways: Exercise, CrossFit, ketogenic diet, low carb nutrition, intermittent fasting, periodic caloric restriction - we know that all these things enhance mitochondrial function.

Things like elevated insulin, glucose, lactate, increased PI3K/AKT/mTOR pathway is a major driver for cancer. There are drugs being developed that target this pathway, by Lew Cantley for example, one of our collaborators. Interestingly, these drugs do not work in the context of a normal diet. They need to be used in the context of a diet that suppresses insulin signaling. So the ketogenic diet dramatically enhances the effect of these metabolically targeted drugs, the PI3 kinase inhibitors.

Elevated ROS and inflammation: So reactive oxygen species overproduction kicks on inflammatory pathways which can damage the mitochondria and really stimulate.

Suppressed anti-tumor immunity: As the tumor pumps out lactate and and lowers the pH, that actually changes the micro environment to prevent your body from recognizing that you have a tumor. And the ketogenic diet increases cancer associated immunity. So it helps increase the vigilance of your immune system to recognize cancer and to attack it through a number of mechanisms. And my colleague Adrienne Scheck, formerly at Barrow Neurological Institute, has studied that and published on that.

So for future directions, we had this idea about an approach for a new cancer treatment approach. And Tom Seyfried, my colleague, we've written and co-authored a review on this. Talking about this idea of a press-pulse approach:

Future Directions for Cancer Therapy

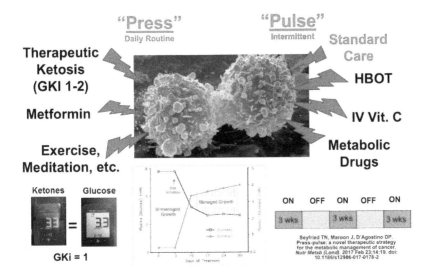

Where a 'press' therapeutic program would be a daily routine of maintaining a high state of therapeutic ketosis.

Dr. Seyfried uses the glucose ketone index [GKi]: If your glucose level is 3 millimolar and your ketone level is 3 millimolar, you would have a glucose ketone index of 1. If your glucose was 4 and your ketones were 2, you would have a glucose ketone index of 2.

We feel that keeping in that 1 to 2 range, if you look at all the animal model studies (especially for seizures), it's extremely therapeutic. It hits all those pathways that I just showed you that target cancer metabolism.

The drug metformin, conceivably, could be used continuously. I think Tom's a little bit resistant against metformin. It may have some side effects.

But exercise, meditation... these things can help you get an ideal glucose-ketone index. Which we know... we talked about the metabolic zone: You bring glucose down to the level of ketones and ketones up.

If you stay within that zone we know experimentally in animal models (and I think the human data will show this and some of it points in that direction) that you are at the very least slowing the tumor, taking the foot off the gas pedal of cancer growth. For the cancers that are responsive to that, that have the Warburg Effect. Or have a 'Warburg phenotype', as we say.

But that sets the stage for other treatment options to be used and our idea is to use them in an on-and-off fashion. Three weeks on, three weeks off.

I am a proponent of standard of care, chemo, radiation and immune therapy. I think for many cancers these can be highly effective and are well tolerated.

I've communicated with enough patients that they get a much better response of these treatments if they're on the ketogenic diet. And they told me the side effects are much less - if they're on the ketogenic diet.

Hyperbaric oxygen therapy [HBOT]: We're just relying on animal model studies now, but... The studies that I showed you from 10 years ago when I was looking at brain tumors, the cells and the mitochondria of the cancer cells were exploding and the normal healthy brain cells were not! I mean, that was very convincing to me that high pressure oxygen was far more toxic to cancer cells than they were to normal healthy cells.

And we published that observation in *Neuroscience* but we really didn't package it as an anti-cancer effect. It was just like an interesting observation.

IV Vitamin C: David Diamond turned me on to this that Vitamin C is a glucose antagonist... Vitamin C at high levels, at millimolar concentration, can be a pro-oxidant! It actually stimulates reactive oxygen species production and oxidative stress.

So it could be used as a pro-oxidant therapy, with or without hyperbaric oxygen therapy. But I think it would work better with hyperbaric oxygen therapy.

And a whole toolbox of metabolic drugs.(...)

Dr. D'Agostinos and Dr. Seyfrieds paper regarding the press-pulse treatment for cancer:

Press-pulse: a novel therapeutic strategy for the metabolic management of cancer
Thomas N. Seyfried, George Yu, Joseph C. Maroon, Dominic P. D'Agostino
Nutr Metab (Lond). 2017 Feb 23

https://pubmed.ncbi.nlm.nih.gov/28250801/

Chapter 3: *Pursuing Health* #97; Interview with Dr. Thomas Seyfried

Introduction & Host Julie Foucher, MD

Hello there and welcome to *Pursuing Health*. This is definitely the most controversial episode of the podcast that I have brought to you to date, but I'm very excited to share this upcoming conversation with you.

A little bit of background about Dr. Seyfried: Thomas Seyfried, PhD, is a biochemical geneticist, scientist and professor at Boston College. For more than 25 years he's taught and conducted research in the fields of neurochemistry, neurogenetics and cancer.

Through his extensive research Thomas has found evidence that supports the hypothesis that cancer is a metabolic disease - as opposed to the mainstream belief that it's genetic in origin.

He believes that this fundamental misunderstanding has led to failed treatment and prevention strategies thus far. In his groundbreaking text *Cancer as a Metabolic Disease* Thomas explains the metabolic theory of cancer step by step, from the most basic science experiments to clinical studies that support this unconventional view.

Now, although it remains unconventional, this metabolic view of the origins of cancer is now shared by many top scientists around the world and is informing their research on metabolic therapies to prevent and treat cancer, including a ketogenic diet.

I think it's important to share the current state of science with patients and with the general public which is why I was so excited to sit down with Dr. Seyfried for this episode.

Science and our conventional dogmas are constantly being challenged, disproven and changing. As one example: Just look at the paradigm shift that's taking place about fat and heart disease over the past several decades.

I highly encourage anyone with a conventional view of cancer to challenge themselves by reading Dr. Seyfried's text before drawing any conclusions of your own.

So Dr. Seyfried and I sat down at the 2018 CrossFit Health Conference (which was held in Madison, Wisconsin) and there we discussed the metabolic theory of cancer, how he came to this understanding and some of the research he's doing on metabolic therapies. As well as some of the challenges that he and others in this research field are facing today.

I really hope that you enjoy this episode, that it will make you think and that it may challenge some of your current views. It certainly did for me.

Foucher:

Welcome to *Pursuing Health!* I'm very excited to be here with Professor Thomas Seyfried who just gave an incredible talk at our CrossFit Health Conference this week. And so thank you for joining me here on the podcast.

Dr. Seyfried:

Thanks Julie, it's nice to be here.

Foucher:

So I thought that we could start with how you got involved with CrossFit becauseI think that's an interesting story in and of itself. How did you end up here at the CrossFit Health Conference?

Dr. Seyfried:

Well, it was Greg Glassman reading my book with his father. And he apparently felt that the argument that I was making in the book was accurate. Having discussed it with his father, reading almost every page. And then I think his father Jeff had a series of issues with some of the data that I presented in the book and he wrote a long series of questions and concerns.

I brought those to my students, my main associate Purna Mukherjee and we discussed it at length. We formulated a rebuttal to Jeff's questions of sufficient detail to appease his concerns. Because I think Greg has a lot of respect for his father, having had a career in precision measurements... and I think that it became clear that what we were saying was accurate, to the best of everyone's ability to understand the information.

And, therefore, contrasted significantly with the standards of what we think cancer is. And I think that kind of overlaps with Greg's philosophy of, iyou know, challenging systems that perpetuate misinformation and I think the cancer field is one of these.

So he became very excited about this. From what I understand he ran around giving everybody... he bought a whole stack of my books and started giving them out to all these CrossFit people.

Foucher:

He did, he gave me one! First time that I had Greg on the podcast he gave me a copy of your book and he gave me a copy of Travis Christofferson's book. And I think he did that for several other people and really got them to read it!

Dr. Seyfried:

Right! So my affiliation with CrossFit came entirely from Greg and his father Jeff. And it wasn't my reaching out to them, they were

60

reaching out to me. Yeah. And I think that he's been a big proponent of our position, let's put it that way. That's spreading the word to a lot of physicians that, you know, maybe...

You heard the the talks that we had here: Jason Fung's discussion was right on, spot on. They're all on... I mean, there are serious problems here and cancer is one of these. I call it 'the big dog' of medicine. I mean, it's just slaughtering people.

You know, type 2 diabetes is not good, it makes you sick and it gives you all these other things. But it doesn't kill you right out. And you don't have to be poisoned! You don't have to believe that you need to get poisened to get a remission or healing. I mean, the whole thing is upside down, it's just crazy.

Foucher:
It is crazy and I want to talk a lot about your work and some of the things you talked about yesterday. But, just to lay the groundwork and the background for people:

Can you describe what your background was in research and how you ended up coming to these conclusions?

Dr. Seyfried:
Yeah. Well, it's a very long and circuitous route, having been trained in lipid biochemistry and genetics. I got my degree in genetics from the University of Illinois and Illinois State University, as well. I have two degrees in genetics, one from Illinois State University and a PhD from the University of Illinois. These are top programs.

But at that time, we were mostly working with gangliosides, it's a lipid molecule that accumulates in the brains of kids with Tay–Sachs disease. So I was studying that, got my PhD in ganglioside biochemistry, trying to look at animal models that had storage disease.

And then I did postdoc at Yale University and then was on the faculty at Yale, in the Department of Neurology. Their big thing there was epilepsy and they were excited about genetics of epilepsy, so we started mapping genes for epilepsy. Because if you want to stay in that department you better do something with epilepsy. So we did epilepsy and gangliosides, epilepsy and genes, epilepsy and this and that.

But here's something interesting: I wrote a proposal to the University at Yale, back in the mid, late 70s. I think it was like '79 or '78, about using ketogenic diet to work with some of the epileptic models. They replied "Oh, that's passe. Nobody does that anymore..."

Foucher:
What prompted you to do that, just because you were looking at previous research?

Dr. Seyfried:
Yeah! I said "Oh, this might be interesting!" But they said "No, no. It's all crap! Diet is not related..."

Foucher:
Interesting.

Dr. Seyfried:
Only later on, when I was at Boston College, one of my students went out to a meeting in Seattle. There was a meeting on epilepsy, basic mechanisms. And Jim Abrams was there. Jim Abrams is a movie producer for Hollywood. He made the *Airplane* movies and the *Naked Gun* movies. You know, those kinds of things.

And and he was pushing keto because his son Charlie was near death from epilepsy.They started the Charlie Foundation. And early on, Meryl Streep (a friend of Jim Abrams) did this *First Do No Harm* movie. Which was about physicians that were pushing drugs onto this kid with epilepsy which was actually Charlie and how it was harming him and killing him.

Jim then found the ketogenic diet by accident at Johns Hopkins and they started putting Charlie on this diet and he did remarkably well. And today, Jim's son Charlie has graduated from college. He's doing really well! I think he may have been married now.

But anyway, Jim was outraged about the system. One of my students heard all this, came back and told me that they're big on this ketogenic diet again. Not again, but she'd never heard of it. I heard of it, of course I knew what it was. But I said "Yale doesn't think anything about that!"

Anyway, we started... she was so enthused, a student of mine. She was so enthusiastic so I said "Alright, we'll try it." This is at Boston College.

Foucher:
So it shows: Enthusiasm can go a long way when you're a student.

Dr. Seyfried:
Yeah. Well, she was very persuasive, "Let's look at it again". But while I was at Yale, I was also doing a lot of lipid research and we were looking at tumors for gangliosides, anyway. That had changed, as one of the people I was working with noted that gangliosides are abnormal

in tumors. So we made some models of brain cancer while I was at Yale and started looking at gangliosides in the brain tumors.

The work was mostly related to the biochemical abnormalities in the tumors. But at the same time we were studying the genetics of epilepsy. So when I left Yale (I took professorship at Boston College) we started to rebuild the whole program from Yale to Boston College.

And we built the animal models, developing more animal models of brain cancer. But at the same time we started ketogenic diets, mapping genes, and then we morphed into using the ketogenic diet for cancer.

However, it started first with doing calorie restriction. Because Dr. Mukherjee joined me in 1999 and she was a big calorie restriction guy. And we actually...

It was very funny, I think it's in Travis's book, too. Because he asked me how I got into this as well. You know, all of these things were going on, but they were not overlapping.

But in our work on gangliosides there was this drug, NBDNJ, that looked like it was impacting Tay–Sachs disease. And I was studying gangliosides, which is the origin of what these lipid storage diseases are.

So by chance, one of my students, myself or somebody... we decided to take this drug and give it to mice that had brain tumors. Just to see if we could change the pattern of gangliosides in the tumor.

Because we had studied gangliosides in tumors, now we were studying Tay–Sachs disease and gangliosides. And my colleague Frances Platt from Oxford University in England had said "Hey, we got this drug, it's really exciting!"

So I had the drug, they sent it to me. And for whatever reason... because, in those days, we had a free animal cost. Now they cost us a fortune! So we were able to do things that we wouldn't do today anymore. Like "Just try it!", didn't write up a protocol, just do it.

And all of a sudden the damn tumors shrunk! On the animals that were being treated it with a ganglioside synthesis inhibitor drug. So I called the company that was making it. Frances, my colleague, told them "Hey, they found this drug could actually shrink tumors!"

So of course now, the company was very interested! Tay–Sachs disease is an orphan disease. It's out of a hundred thousand people one gets this disease. It's a devastating disease to the kids. I mean, let's be honest. And we're still working on it, by the way.

But, of course the company "Oh wow!" - because cancer is massively bigger than Tay–Sachs disease. So they heard that I had found that this ganglioside drug shrunk tumors. So they asked me "How much money do you need? Just tell me the check and I'll write it out, because we want you to explore this!" So I said "Hm, maybe 200,000 dollars." "Not

63

a problem!" They gave me the $200,000 immediately! It was like the next day the check came in to the University for my research.

So we started then more detailed analysis of the drug. And sure enough, we give the mice to drug and they would eat the food...but we noticed that their body weights were getting smaller, okay? In fact, I hired Purna to help me with this drug work because she had been doing a lot of animal work with calorie restriction and all this stuff.

So she came in and said "The drug has an anti-angiogenic effect!" - which is even more powerful, which is more exciting. It shrinks blood vessels and all this. But we all noticed that the animals that were eating the drug, their body weights were getting lower.

But then somebody said "Well, you got to be really careful about some of these drugs because they induce an indirect calorie restriction!"

So I said "Okay, let's set up a new experiment: We're going to have
- Animals that get no drug - their tumors grow like crazy. (Group 1)
- Animals that get the drug - their tumors are much smaller. (Group 2)
- And a third group: Animals that don't get the drug but restricted food to equal the body weight of the drug group. (Group 3)

And the results of group 2 and 3 came out exactly the same! So the drug had actually no effect on anything other than the fact that it made the mice eat less food! And their body weights shrunk and that was all an indirect calorie restriction effect.

Foucher:
The company probably wasn't too excited about that!

Dr. Seyfried:
Yes, they were quite livid! So they tried to tell me that "Well, when you write it up you got to just focus on the change of the gangliosides in the tumor because that's what's going to be exciting!" Yes, the drug did change gangliosides in the tumor. But that wasn't the therapeutic effect. That wasn't why it was working. It was working because it induced calorie restriction.

And then we went on to show later on, that calorie restriction lowers blood sugar and elevates ketones. Then we fell back on Warburg who found the same thing many years before us.

I said "What's going on here?" It works, because the calorie restriction lowers blood sugar. Warburg said sugars are driving the tumors and they have a defective respiration.

So when we published the paper they said, "Don't put the calorie restriction stuff in there!" and I said that I had to do it. "I'm not gonna lie, this is the main part!" They were upset about it, of course, and they pulled the plug. No more money. Because we actually had found a mechanism that wasn't sexy, basically.

Foucher:
Wasn't gonna make them any money.

Dr. Seyfried:
No, this was not going to make them any money - when you can get the same effect by eating less food, you know! So they dumped us on that.

Foucher:
So you had then found out more about Warburg's work through this?

Dr. Seyfried:
Yeah. Well, at the time I did not know too much. I had heard of him, everybody heard of Warburg. Warburg is just his name, *Warburg*, because he built the apparatus. Like, it's just the *Warburg machine* the *Warburg* this and that. And he had been a major figure. But, you know, as a geneticist and as a lipid biochemist in epilepsy and gangliosides, Warburg's work never really came into our research at all. But when we found out aboutthe glucose stuff...

Linda Nebeling (whose work I referenced) did a paper in 1995: She treated little kids with brain cancer based on Warburg's theory of lowering blood sugar and elevating ketones.

Warburg didn't talk too much about ketones but he certainly talked about blood sugar. So we were seeing the same thing in these mice that were getting the so called 'special drug', that was lowering blood sugar and elevating ketones. And I said "Well, that's just what we use ketogenic diets for: To lower blood sugar and elevate ketones in the kids to stop their seizures."

I said "This drug is doing the same thing and stopping the growth of the tumor!" Warburg said "It's all because the cancer cells have damaged respiration." So we went back and looked at Warburg's hypothesis and theory very carefully and we said "Warburg! This guy's probably right"

Foucher:
And can you explain for people listening who aren't familiar what his theory is and how that differs from our current conventional conception?

Dr. Seyfried:
Well, Warburg made the seminal discovery that all cancer cells produce large amounts of lactic acid. And that's confirmed over and over again, everywhere. And the PET scans, fluorodeoxyglucose-PET scans, light up tumors because they're sucking down so much glucose. But they're also blowing out lactic acid.

And Louis Pasteur in the 1800s made the fundamental discovery that yeast cells are fermenting. They produce a lot of lactic acid. But as soon as oxygen comes in, they stop fermenting and they respire. They don't produce lactic acid anymore, with oxygen. And that's called the Pasteur Effect. And Warburg had mentioned this Pasteur Effect and he argued the cancer cells have a defective Pasteur Effect.

Because even if you put oxygen into the environment, unlike the yeast, the cancer cell continues to make lactic acid even though the oxygen is present. So, clearly, deviating from what Louis Pasteur had said. And Warburg said "Well, how do you explain that? Why would a cancer cell continue to ferment when oxygen is present?" And he put these cancer cells in 100% oxygen and they still made lactic acid, which is incredible!

He came to the major conclusion that their respiration is defective. And the reason why they have to ferment is because they can't respire. He went through elegant experiments, one after another, looking at normal tissues, cancer tissues, all kinds of stuff. And he came to this conclusion that respiration is defective and that's the reason why they ferment.

A lot of people today, even today, don't believe that! They think Warburg was wrong. Only because if Warburg is right almost everybody else is wrong! So they have to defend the status quo by saying Warburg is wrong - with minimal information or misinformation about his theory. That's going on today from some of the top medical schools, arguing that Warburg was wrong.

I wrote the book to prove that Warburg was in fact right! And I went through massive amounts of data, from hundreds of experiments, over decades of research. From electron microscopy, protein chemistry, lipid chemistry, everything.

We have done research in our lab to show that respiratory systems in mouse tumors are defective - no question about it! And that's the reason they ferment, exactly supporting Warburg's theory. And yet, people ignore all this.

66

It's too devastating to say that this guy, Warburg (who had won the Nobel Prize) was right. He was kind of an arrogant German scientist... he was spared by Hitler because Hitler feared cancer and Warburg was the leading cancer guy in the world. Even though he was part jew. Hitler said "I determine who is jew and not jew!"

Because he decided this guy's could save his life, possibly. If Germany had won the war, cancer probably would have been cured! Of course, everything with Germany after the war was just discredited.

Foucher:
So is that why this theory got kind of pushed aside?

Dr. Seyfried:
It got pushed aside for several reasons. Number one: There had been always a debate about the origin of the lactic acid. Was it really damaged respiration? A lot of experiments that weren't done correctly said it wasn't. Other experiments that were done correctly said it was.

But at the same time Watson and Crick had discovered the structure of DNA. And then they found that there were DNA abnormalities in tumor cells. This was the sexy and hottest thing in science in the 20th century - and everybody ran off chasing genes! And it stayed that way and today we're still suffering from that migration, that lemmings-kind of groupthink migration.

Because the DNA discovery was so profound... we discovered the defects at the molecular origin of the gene. The gene is DNA and the genes control everything and genes are defective, DNA is defective in tumors.

Foucher:
So maybe all this is just about the timing of these discoveries.

Dr. Seyfried:
What happened was: All the biochemists, everybody ran after the genetic defects in cancer and felt that this was the origin of the disease. It even goes back to early 20th century, when Boveri found abnormal chromosomes in cancers and said "Oh, this is probably the origin!"

But even the pathologists said that that was all secondary downstream effects, these chromosomes. And there had been many other papers in the literature saying it's got to be some mitochondrial thing, it can't be genetic. But, you know, everybody was swept away with the DNA and the genes.

And then they started giving Nobel Prizes out to people who were finding oncogenes and tumor suppressor genes and this kind of stuff. Everybody likes to go with the crowd, guys that think they know everything and the whole fields has morphed into this chasing genes thing.

Foucher:
I think you did a great job in your talk this week of illustrating the difference of your approach compared to the prevailing theory to date:

That it's the DNA damage and the nucleus that's driving cancer - versus your metabolic explanation where this is all starting in the mitochondria. And that that's later causing the nuclear damages as a result.

Dr. Seyfried:
That's right. What I did was I rearranged the players in the cancer field and simply showed that all the gene mutations are coming from damage to the respiration. Which produce reactive oxygen species, which are mutagenic. So, basically, the mutations are an effect and not the cause!

So the whole thing, "Where does cancer come from?" becomes much more explainable. It comes from damaged respiration. Exactly as Warburg said. The problem is Warburg didn't know about all of the other ways that cells could get energy without respiration. And we're doing that now.

We're filling in the missing parts of Warburg's central theory, finding the missing link. Which then should resolve all the controversy. Once that happens, then we know exactly where cancer comes from, how it comes and how we can treat it. And that's gonna be a big thing.

The problem is - as we've heard at this meeting - revenue generation seems to be more important than patient health. If we put revenue generation as the prime goal of this and disease management and patient health as a secondary goal, then we're never going to get to the promised land of reducing cancer.

So this is the thing that physicians have to do. They can't be just simply drug pushers for the pharmaceutical industry and I think we heard about that problem here at this meeting. But a lot of physicians allow themselves to become that. Not that they want to become that, but...

Foucher:
...it's just what the system does.

Dr. Seyfried:
It's what the system forces them to do. And once you're in the system... unlike me. I'm not in the system. So I can say what the hell I

68

want to say because I don't have a medical license to lose. But my friends who are in the system, if they try to do what we think we shoud be doing, they're reprimanded. Or could potentially lose their license for practicing medicine that is not sanctioned by the establishment.

And if you're going to cure cancer, you've got to stop doing the nonsense that the establishment says you should do. Okay? So all this radiation and chemo and all this kind of stuff, you don't need to do a lot of that. You can manage these diseases without toxicity and cost effective.

But, you know, the system is so powerful! It creates... for some physicians, they just have to ignore the truth. You just can't accept the reality that the treatments that you're giving to your patients are actually counterproductive to their health and wellbeing. And you just have to say "I'm doing it because Big Brother told me to do it."

But then there's those physicians that have a moral conscience. They have to be torn immensely within their soul, knowing that what they're actually doing is harmful. And they know that what they're doing is not good. And they also know that there is another way they could treat their patients and they're not allowed to do that! It has to be terribly frustrating for these poor people.

Foucher:
Do you think that there are a lot of physicians who know that? Or do you think that there are a lot of people who just don't see the other solution?

Dr. Seyfried:
I think it's a combination of both. But I think the majority never heard of what we're saying. When you get into the practice of medicine, the practice of your art, you just have so many patients and you have to do so many time consuming things and you're just doing all that. You don't have time to sit down and read the literature to determine whether or not what you're doing is right.

However, it becomes even more difficult because there are many physicians that have the opportunity to do some basic research as part of their internship or residency or whatever the hell they want to call it, it's always confusing to me. But they have that opportunity.

And that's where some of them actually say "Hey, this is not right!" But then when they take it to the higher-ups, those say "Oh, Warburg was wrong!" And if you do that you could potentially lose your grant and you could potentially have a lot of problems. So people don't want to do that.

Foucher:
It's too controversial.

Dr. Seyfried:
Yeah, because you're against the major... The so-called hot thing in cancer today is immunotherapies. You see them advertised on TV in the evening, Keytruda, Opdivo.

Now we even have CAR-T immunotherapies being advertised on TV. Which is an abomination because it hasn't been proven, it kills as many people as it could help! But yet people don't hear that! They only hear what the establishment wants them to hear. And you heard that from Dr. Revins today!

If you have anything that goes against the Big Brother then you will not be heard. It's just that simple. So what is the common person supposed to know? They say "Look at the advances in cancers, we get all these wonderful treatments!" Until they are the ones that have to take the treatment. And then they're asking "How come, it didn't work the way you told me it was? And I had to pay $400,000!"

Foucher:
And you also showed some data at the very beginning of your talk about the increasing death rates with cancer, despite all those efforts.

Dr. Seyfried:
Yeah! And as I said, why nobody knows about this? I mean, this is common knowledge! The American Cancer Society blogs this information every year. But nobody reads it! They all think cancer is... that we're managing cancer real well. But then you look around and see the truth!

And as I said in my book: All you have to do is read the obituary page in any newspaper and you're going to ask yourself "Why all these people dying from cancer?" If we have a solution and it's working why is the obituary page full of people dying from cancer? Makes no sense! It's common sense that it's not working.

And you saw the death statistics: 1,600 people a day dying from cancer? Over 1,600 people - and it's getting worse every year!

Now, if you do metabolic therapy the way we think we should do it, we would drop that death rate by 50% in 10 years!

Which would be enormous, right? Think about it! 50 percent of lives saved that are being currently lost because of a misunderstanding of the nature of the disease. So if you look at... what's pushing the CAR T-Cell therapy, these immunotherapies, is the genes theory of cancer.

70

So if the gene theory of cancer is wrong (like we showed in our nuclear transfer experiments, I put them all together) then the very therapies that they're telling us will work are not going to work! They do work for a few people, okay? Just by, I don't know, maybe by chance or something. But most people don't respond the way they're supposed to respond. And oftentimes, they can get killed from this. It can kill them!

No physician should ever administer a therapy to a patient where there's a remote chance that this therapy could kill the patient. Or significantly harm them. But they do this!

Foucher:
That's cancer treatment, right?

Dr. Seyfried:
Yeah. But why? Why are they doing this? Because they say "We have to stop the growing cells." We showed that the growing cells need two fuels, glucose and glutamine. If you take them away the growing cells will die. That's so much easier!

Foucher:
Can you talk more about that, about the glutamine and about filling in some of these gaps from Warburg's research? And where you're at in leading into this metabolic treatment?

Dr. Seyfried:
Well, we all know the cancer cells are sucking down glucose. But there are some tumors that don't take in very much glucose and they grow like crazy. So therefore Warburg must be wrong.

But they're fermenting a different molecule, they're not using sugar to do lactic acid fermentation. They're using glutamine to do succinic acid fermentation. This is an amino acid fermentation and it's been well known. A lot of microorganisms do this kind of stuff. But the cancer cell falls back in doing the same thing.

So basically, they're not respiring, can't get energy from respiration. That's why they live in hypoxic environments. They can live without oxygen and this is what Warburg showed. You take the oxygen away, the cancer cells survive. Normal cells die.

Nobody can live without oxygen - but cancer cells can! You can give cancer cells cyanide. Cyanide kills people! Cancer cells are resistant to cyanide!

Foucher:
They'll be fine.

Dr. Seyfried:
Yeah, right! So when you put that... cancer cells can live in cyanide, that's what we're talking about! You know, nobody can live without oxygen but cancer cells can because they don't respire, they ferment! And cyanide attacks respiration, it doesn't attack fermentation. So if Warburg is wrong, how come the cancer cell can live in cyonide?

Foucher:
Interesting!

Dr. Seyfried:
People ignore all this. Because it's too difficult to accept the fact that Warburg was right. And then you have to go back and say "Everything that I'm doing is wrong - and I can prove it because we get all these dead people. And if they're not dead, they're seriously damaged from what I did to them."

Now they have to be treated for diabetes management, there are psychiatric problems, hormonal imbalances, gut and digestive issues. You can name it, go on. On and on.

So we have a new branch of medicine called 'cancer survivor' medicine. "Oh wow, we have another whole bunch of people remaining in the system that we can continue to treat with anti-diabetic drugs..." and all the things that we heard here that they're all bullshit.

Anyway, the whole thing... and I agree: I think CrossFit's idea that there's a mess, is understated. It's a big mess!

Foucher:
It is a big mess! I think the more you learn about it, the bigger you realize it is.

Dr. Seyfried:
Yeah.

Foucher:
So for the glutamine, is that something that is consistent across all types of cancer?

Dr. Seyfried:
I think so. I think to one degree or another... not all, because there are some (very few) that don't use any glutamine. It's all glucose dependent. So you take a cancer that's completely glucose dependent, they should be really powerfully impacted by ketogenic diets. A ketogenic diet and lowering blood sugar will demolish these tumors.

But then, the ketogenic diet doesn't work against tumors that are heavily glutamine dependent. So there's where you got to target the glutamine. And if you target the glutamine and the glucose together... we don't think there's any tumor cell that can survive in the absence of these two fuels!

Foucher:
You think those are the only two fuels out there that cancer cells can run on?

Dr. Seyfried:
They can run on other amino acids and small carbs, but there's not enough. If you're going to run a train you got to have a sufficient amount of material. You got to have sufficient sufficient fuel. And if you don't have enough fuel... the cells burn it up real quick and then they run out of fuel. Again, when they run out of fuel, they die!

So you have to have what we call 'logistics': It's the supply of the cancer cell. So there has to be a sufficient supply of the fermentable fuel to keep the beast going. Glucose and glutamine are the only two fuels that are present in massive quantities that would allow this. All the other fuels that could be used could be sucked down in about a day or two.

Foucher:
Okay. There's not enough of them.

Dr. Seyfried:
Yeah, the cancer cell can ferment other amino acids, like aspartate, any of these amino acids. But some of these amino acids, to be fermented, you also have to spend energy to get them into the fermentable state. So to get energy you're spending energy. Glutamine requires no energy expenditure, it's a pure fuel. Just like glucose.

So those two are pure fuels, they require very little other energy. They give you more ATP than they consume. Whereas other amino acid fermentations can take equal amounts for what they yield. And they're not present in sufficient quantity, whereas glutamine is the most abundant amino acid in the body and it can be synthesized from glucose.

So if you take away glucose, you can't synthesize glutamine. If you take away glutamine, you can't drive the tumor. If you take the two of them away, the tumor can't survive. It's just that simple!

Foucher:

And are there certain types of cancers that you know of that are higher in their ability to use glutamine?

Dr. Seyfried:

Yes, there are. There are some cancers that don't show up on PET scan and we asked ourselves what was going on. And they're sucking taking down glutamine! So a lot of the immune cells system cancers are sucking glutamine down big time. Like a lot of the leukemias, myeloids, these kinds of things.

Foucher:

The ketogenic diet probably wouldn't work as well, with those cancers?

Dr. Seyfried:

It works. It works but because it reduces inflammation. It does a lot of other things that provoke... but I think to kill them off big time, you got to target both molecules. So there's a checkmate: You can't move into that spot, you can't move into this spot - you're dead!

So... and who's doing that? No one! We're the only group that actually tried to do this! We did it on a brain cancer patient with good success.

Foucher:

Can you talk about that? About your metabolic therapy and the press-pulse?

Dr. Seyfried:

Yeah. Well, the press-pulse was developed from a concept of paleobiology. People who study the history of the earth knew that in the past there were these massive extinctions of organisms on the planet. And then they would evolve into a new group of organisms.

So they were going back and saying "What was responsible for these mass extinctions of organisms?" And there were two unlikely events that coincided, basically some sort of stress, like a climate change or something like this, that was putting stress on the population.

Some individuals of the population were dying because they couldn't handle the stress, others were adapting to the stress and surviving, but under difficult situations. And then, all of a sudden, like a series of volcanic explosions or a meteorite strike, together with this climate 'press', led to the complete extermination of all organisms.

So you can see where we're going with this: If we develop a therapy that 'presses' the entire body, where cancer cells are under greater stress than the normal cells and then we bring in drugs to 'pulse'... and the pulsing drugs:

We protect the whole body with ketones and put the patients into a good physiological state that kills a lot of tumor cells but won't kill the glutamine ones.

And then we pulse with other drugs that put even greater pressure on both glucose and glutamine, while the body is under the press. This is the strategy. So it's press-pulse.

And what happens is that the patients emerge from the therapy healthier than than when they started! And oftentimes what we see of these patients is: Not only do they have cancer, they have all these other abnormalities! They have vitamin deficiencies, they have diabetes, they have all kinds of other things. All that stuff goes away, along with the tumor!

Foucher:
They get more than they've bargained for!

Dr. Seyfried:
Oh, you get a lot more than you bargained for. It's unbelievable. And they don't have hair loss and bleeding and they don't have vomiting and all this kind of crap. So you can actually destroy the tumor gradually using press-pulse therapeutic strategy. The goal is to gradually degrade the tumor.

As a matter of fact - because glutamine is such a powerful and important metabolite for our body - you can't just take away glutamine and not expect to have other toxic events. So what we do is:

While we're in the process, we'll hit them with the glutamine drug and immediately give them glutamine. Or even give them glutamine, while the drug. Or even before we give the drug!

Foucher:
Ah, interesting.

Dr. Seyfried:
Because our immune system needs the glutamine. So if I kill a whole cartload of tumor cells, our immune system has to come in and pick up the corpses. And if our immune system is paralyzed and can't pick up the corpses... (even though the immune system is not dead, it's just paralyzed from taking the glutamin drugs) but the immune system needs glutamine to do its job!

So you can't just expect... if you kill the cancer cells and nobody picks them up, you get tumorlysis, you get all kinds of other infections! You have to do it strategically. So you want to kill a whole bunch of cells and then you want to bring the same molecule that you just took away. Give it back (because the immune system needs it) they'll come in and pick up all the dead bodies, clear up the system - and then hit the cancer again!

So even though you give them back a little glutamine, you've already cut the tumor population in half. That's good. You've got them under the press so even if they have their glutamine, they're not gonna be able to grow real fast.

So only a few of them will grow but then you're gonna hit the cancer, the glutamin metabolism again and *boom*, another 25-30 percent of them are gone. And then you get maybe another 5% growing back, and hit him again, *boom* another big part is going to die! Eventually, the cancer calles are gone! Right? And it's beautiful!

And each grade that you give, each position, the patients are getting healthier and healthier: They're getting healthier because their tumors are going away - and they're getting healthier because a lot of the other covariables get better!

Foucher:
Inflammation, metabolic diseases in general...

Dr. Seyfried:
Yeah, all these other diseases that they had are also being managed at the same time! So it's a win-win situation for the patient. But not for the traditional medicine! Which is... we should never be poisoning and radiating people to make them healthy in the first place.

And then we put the patients into hyperbaric oxygen chambers which acts as a surrogate for radiation. It kills the tumor cell by oxidative stress. And we heat them up, sometimes. We can heat up tissue which puts more oxidative stress on the tumor cells.

There's so many new ways that we can kill tumor cells. It becomes... you can get giddy thinking about this because you say "Oh, let me try that! Does that work with this? Yeah, it works even better! Wow!"

Foucher:
So many new combinations.

Dr. Seyfried:
Yes! And I think if a physician understood this, their philosophy of treating patients would just be so exciting. It would be almost like a CrossFit competition: You could say to somebody "Do you know how easy I could kill those cancer cells if you do this, on this regimen, instead of that? Now, watch this!"

This is super exciting!

76

And nobody's doing this because they think it's a genetic disease!

So they build all these absurd things that make people sick and kill them. And it doesn't help the majority of the patients.

Foucher:
It costs a lot of money.

Dr. Seyfried:
Yes, it costs a ton of money, it's just... it's incredible. So I think that the future of cancer is so bright. But at the same time so dim. And that's the tragedy. We just have to get rid of this nonsense. And CrossFit may be one of the ways to do this. It's just amazing to say that, but it's possible. It could happen!

Because if it can withstand the storm that will come... and believe me, you saw how powerful the contrary views are. But I think Greg and the power of the CrossFit community could make a difference. They would need to be part of the spearhead, the tip of the spear to crack this absurdity in cancer that we call "standard of care".

Foucher:
I think we're just starting to see it. This week is just the very tip of the iceberg of what CrossFit is doing. And it's similar to... we've heard Gary Taubes speak as well, about the paradigm shift in fat, the 'calories-in calories-out' theory. And he started writing about that 15 years ago! And now we're finally at a place, where that stuff is going to change.

Dr. Seyfried:
But the general public still doesn't understand that.

Foucher:
Yeah, there's still so many people who don't understand it. But at least the medical community is starting to wrap their heads around it. And, you know, nutrition recommendations are changing.

Dr. Seyfried:
Yes, I agree.

Foucher:
The change is slow. Much slower than we would all like.

Dr. Seyfried:

Yeah and I think we heard today about the nonsense of statin drugs. And don't forget: Not long ago, it's just a couple years ago, there was some guy (can't remember his name) who said that everybody who reaches 50 years of age should start on statin drugs! Whether they have any disease or not!

Foucher:

So can you talk a little bit about your research? I know in your lab you focus mostly on mice, right? Mice models...

Dr. Seyfried:

Yeah.

Foucher:

...but I know that you work with physicians all over the world in different groups who are implementing or have implemented your press-pulse therapy in patients.

So can you just talk about where we're at in that stage? And then maybe about some of the challenges to being able to implement this on a larger scale with humans?

Dr. Seyfried:

Well, I think where we have less rigidity... and I'm just saying less, not no. Because everywhere we go, we're locked by this absurdity of the standard of care. And therefore we have to modify it.

We can do modifications easier in some other clinics that we can in in the so-called 'westernized clinics' where you don't have any leeway. It's written in stone and granite and you can't change it. At least, so far, we can't change it.

But when we go to other places, we can modify it. And when we modify it, bringing in metabolic therapy, I think the results are so much more positive and so much more remarkable.

Foucher:

When you're saying using metabolic therapy, do you mean metabolic therapy alone or in conjuction with other therapies?

Dr. Seyfried:

So far we have not been able to use metabolic therapy alone. In any clinic. We've always been yoked by having to use some standard of care. Because everybody has become so brainwashed to think that standard of care or some aspect of standard of care is still good.

78

In my view it's all bunk! Because the purpose of standard of care is kill tumour cells. And if you can kill tumor cells without toxicity why would you want to use anything that has toxicity associated with it? But they can't accept that, they don't know about it, they don't understand. It's not that complicated!

I mean, if lay people can understand it, more conclusively than the professionals, what does that say? I mean... right?

Foucher:
Professionals often overcomplicate things.

Dr. Seyfried:
Well, even if they're not overcomplicating it, they can't. They're not allowed to. Okay? They're restricted in what they're capable of doing.

And then when people argue "Oh, this metabolic therapy hasn't been proven!" Well, it's been proven at the basic science level. Unquestionably! The basic science says that this is the way to do it! The preclinical systems say this is the way to do it. The only people who are not doing it is in the clinical systems because they say "It hasn't been vetted by a clinical trial!"

Okay. So when you do a clinical trial on a metabolic therapy, it's very very difficult to get anybody to do it. And if they do allow it to be done, it's got to be some stage four terminal cancer when the patient's already been beat to hell by drugs, by radiation and chemo.

And then we're going to take them and then we're going to try to rally all their body, to try recover from all the damage that you've already done to it... oh, and besides: Trying to manage this now outrageously growing cancer that was created by the very standards of care!

So now you're expecting this metabolic therapy to correct everything...

Foucher:
A tall order.

Dr. Seyfried:
... a tall order. But in fact it can be done in some cases. But the bigger issue, as I mentioned: We can't do the critical control group. That's not allowed. It's taboo, but the critical control group would have to be a metabolic therapy *without* standard of care.

What would happen if the metabolic therapy without standard of care is superior to both standard of care and the combination of metabolic therapy with standard of care? Metabolic therapy by itself trumps out chemotherapy, radiation therapy and immunotherapy. Beats them all! Right? What would happen?

Foucher:
Yeah, then we'd have a great problem for our current industry.

Dr. Seyfried:
I know exactly what's going to happen: These people are going to do a hell of a lot better! You saw Pablo Kelly! He's only one of many, you know. They're rejecting standard of care and they're surviving!

Now, you don't go and do nothing. Standard of care is still better than eating big jelly donuts. But if you don't eat the jelly donuts and you do metabolic therapy you're going to trump standard of care. I have no doubt about it, it I've seen it work. It's just unbelievable.

So, we just have to get physicians that understand...

Number one: Understand. And number two: Are allowed to practice what they should be doing. And if you don't understand it and you're not allowed to do it, you're not going to do it.

Foucher:
Right. So it sounds like today most of the experience with this is just in individuals who say "I don't want to do the standard of care and I want to try this instead!" And it can't be part of a traditional research study per se because you're not allowed to forego the standard of care in research.

Dr. Seyfried:
Yeah. But when we do standard of care in brain cancer, we see that everybody who gets radiation dies. Over and over again. Everything you see, people are getting standard of care, 98% of all the people are dead within six years. That's solid data. Nobody's gonna argue with that because it's been repeated thousands and thousands of times.

And you come along and you get a guy who decides not to do this and he lives much longer than you would expect. They still say "Well, we can't consider him at all because he's not part of a clinical trial."

But you still have a few functional brain cells! So if you're the patient, you can say "What the hell? How could that guy survive so long? I want to do what he's doing!" Right? "Maybe it will work! And what about this guy? Did the same thing, he's doing well! And what about that guy over there?"

Still, the establishment is going to say "Well, we can't consider those because they're not part of a clinical trial." "So what? They're alive and they have good quality of life. I want to do what they're doing! I don't give a shit about the clinical trial!" You know. It's just common sense!

80

And besides cancer: People want to live! I mean, this is not some incidental thing, nobody goes "Well, I'll put it off...", you know. No no. Cancer patients are going to demand "I want to do what those guys are doing so I can stay alive!" And then you go to your physician and you say "Hey, I don't want all that standard of care, cause it could harm me!"

And one of the things we don't know... I haven't seen any statistics on this, yet: Of the people who take standard of care and die, it's not clear how many people are dying from the disease or from the treatments. That has always been a mystery. Because we don't know.

Doctors say "He was treated aggressively... and then he died." Well, how do we know that it was the cancer? Because there are so many radical remissions of cancer in people who don't take standard of care!

And Kelly Turner did this book, *Radical Remissions*. There were a lot of things that were associated with those remissions, but one of the things was radical changes in diet. That was one of the things that was most common in people who had radical cancer remission. A radical change in diet! Oh, does that say something?

Foucher:
Yeah, interesting.

Dr. Seyfried:
Right? But as a physician in the system you're not allowed to consider that. Because it hasn't been vetted. And those double-blind crossovers that are required for standard of care, or to put a new therapy into place, this setup is designed to keep the status quo.

The requirements are designed to only allow another drug to replace a drug that's already there. Not a completely different system. Not a completely different paradigm of treating cancer.

Because there's no way to know if our therapy is the best treatment when those studies can't be done! Our guy's not eating for three days, he's in an hyperbaric chamber, he's eating fat when he does eat.

It's completely impossible to get those studies done without the standard of care stuff! You just have to say based on the hard science, the preclinical studies, the case reports that are published: "We should just do it!"

Foucher:
Let's just do it!

Dr. Seyfried:
Yeah, let's just do it! And have the appropriate control groups. The only group we can't have is the 'know-nothing group'. Okay? We can't just not treat people. So, we have

- the standard of care (which we have massive evidence for)
- metabolic therapy combined with the standard of care. And then we have
- metabolic therapy by itself.

So that kind of a controlled study would solve this problem. That would give us the data that would tell us which treatment is better. Now, who's gonna pay for that?

Foucher:
Right, who's gonna pay for that and also, again, being a vulnerable population, people who are diagnosed with cancer and, like you said, are very desperate to try anything that will work. That poses some challenges as well.

Dr. Seyfried:
Yeah. But when you look at all the things up until now: Nothing has worked!

Foucher:
Yeah.

Dr. Seyfried:
The patients are not told that. They're just told "This is the new drug, we got something new. It could work," you know.

But all the other hundreds of drugs didn't work. Almost nothing that's come out of the genome sequencing has worked. The evidence that the treatment you're going to get is not going to work is overwhelming! Right? Well, we have all this other stuff on metabolic therapy that shows that these people can do really well. Why would you not want to take that?

The turkish group, they only take stage four cancers, so-called "terminal cancers" and keeping these people alive for much, much longer - at a higher quality of life. And with some people it maybe even resolved! You can't know, because it's just been recent, we haven't started this up until recently.

You've got to wait 10, 12 years to know. If the guy is alive and he's doing well and he has no adverse effects from the treatments and he's doing fine, then you get more and more of these people. The ex-patients will get on the web and say "Hey, if you do this, you're gonna survive!"

All of a sudden the patient's gonna come to the physician and say "Thank you, but I want the metabolic therapy."

"We don't do that."

"What the hell! I'm gonna go somewhere where they do it. I'm gonna go to CrossFit, they do it over there!"

Foucher:
That's right. And I know you get emails all the time from people who have a cancer diagnosis. Or maybe there's people listening who just recently had a cancer diagnosis and they are hearing this and they're wondering "Where do I go from here? What should I do?"

Dr. Seyfried:
Well, I send them a kit with information on glucose-ketone index calculators. Because a person... just like Jason Fung was telling, the power is in your hand. If you can get yourself into therapeutic ketosis, you're on the right step. Okay?

Then once you're there, you can think about your next step. But you kind of have the physician to move you to the next step... you can't just put your ass into a hyperbaric oxygen chamber. Well, actually that's not completely true. There are people who are renting them for their homes.

Foucher:
Oh, really?

Dr. Seyfried:
They get in there, they tighten it up and they turn the gas on, or have somebody in the family turn the gas on.

Foucher:
Wow!

Dr. Seyfried:
But you'd like to be in a professional setting to do hyperbaric oxygen. And the problem is that they're not generally part of the treatment.

Here's another bizarre thing: If you get irradiated for cancer treatment and your gut is all damaged and your body is all damaged, the insurance company will pay for you to have hyperbaric oxygen to repair the damage from the radiation therapy. But they will not allow to use hyperbaric oxygen therapy to kill the cancer!

Foucher:
Hm. Not approved yet.

Dr. Seyfried:
Approved for what? Why? What do you ned an approval for, you're gonna take the same therapy?

Foucher:
Right, right.
Except, if you do it before you take the radiation, you don't have to take the radiation!

Foucher:
The irony...

Dr. Seyfried:
I know!
So physicians have to rally. They have to form a physicians organization that stands up to this absurdity. I'm not saying the standard of care is absurd in all cases. Of course, there are some diseases where standard of care is in fact the best, there is no other option.

But in cancer, and in particular type 2 diabetes and these kinds of things... well, I say more 'chronic disease management', this is where metabolic therapies will have the biggest impact.

But you're standing... as I said in my talk, you got the 800-pound gorilla that sits in the room that is basically Big Pharma - and the federal US federal government that's sleeping in bed with the gorilla!

And that is a big obstacle to move. Because the firestorm that comes back, to say... they've called them "merchants of doubt". There's a book *Merchants of Doubt,* the guys who claim that this climate change doesn't exist and all this kind of stuff.... or tobacco doesn't harm you, you know.

They find a study where it's shown that this guy who smoked tobacco never got hurt or whatever... and it creates doubt on the part of the people to say "Well, maybe they're not completely right." So those people will come in and show some guy who does metabolic therapy and doesn't respond - where thousand of others did.

The general public is going to say "Well, maybe most people won't respond to that treatment". And this is going to be a planned undermining of the message.

Because there's organizations that have too much to lose if this now changes.

But, you know, as I said: The bottom line is that people want to live, they want to be treated without toxicity. I can tell you now, in cancer: If you get cancer, I don't know if they fear the disease more than the treatment! Because they feel like "I'm gonna have to lose my breasts, my hair's gonna fall out! My face!"

I mean, to people who are interested in their personal appearance this is devastating!

Foucher:
Yeah, and let alone how you feel. You're feeling weak all the time.

Dr. Seyfried:
Yeah, you're sick all the time. Fatigue, nausea. Your hair is falling out, you're gonna get your breasts removed, your colon cut out. I mean, this is like... give me a break!

"I got to be on Imodium for the rest of my life, I got to carry a colostomy bag. I'm gonna lose my arm! My whole life will change!"

Foucher:
Not a good situation.

Dr. Seyfried:
No! It's devastating! Completely devastating! I put a lot of that in my book in the first chapter. About what it means to have cancer and all these different images. You can look at it as a genetic disorder and look at a whole bunch of gene mutations - and nobody gets freaked out looking at a whole bunch of little spots or graphs, right?

But when you see a woman with a mastectomy, no hair and all this kind of stuff then you start to see the real impact of what the hell is going on.

Foucher:
Yeah, and what it does to your family and your financial situation and all of those other things.

Dr. Seyfried:
Yeah, that's terrible. And with the new push on the immunotherapies... it's funny that the ones that work best, the people who respond best are the ones to get the highest fever. This has been shown on a number of occasions.

And William Coley did that many years ago when he gave live bacteria to his cancer patients. They got Staph and Strep and of course, that's going to cause a response you get from sepsis: Your body goes into a massively high fever, 103, 104 maybe even higher. Right on the precipice of death.

But if you can survive the fever your cancer is completely destroyed. And he was able to cure a lot of people with advanced cancer, just by raising the body temperature with a bacterial infection. Then they changed it from live bacteria to killed bacteria and gave it to the patients.

And of course their body responded as if the bacteria were alive and they had the high fever and it worked just as well. But they get rid of that because the 5% of the people had fevers they couldn't control and died.

But it's interesting that the immunotherapies that you give today for $350,000, you'll do best if you get a high fever. And the patients who don't do as well don't get the high fever! So what is this "new treatment" after all? It's a Coley vaccine all over again!

Foucher:
Very interesting, wow!

Dr. Seyfried:
Haha! And Coley didn't charge anything for his vaccine!

Foucher:
Free bacteria.

Dr. Seyfried:
Yeah.

Foucher:
Okay, so maybe we'll start wrapping up, but can you give us just an overview of where this field of research is? The things that you're working on, are there maybe other like-minded researchers or people who are working on this metabolic therapy as well? Where are we at in this country and around the world? Where do we have to go next?

Dr. Seyfried:
Well, I think the biggest thing is:
You got to convince people that this is a metabolic disease. It's a mitochondrial metabolic disease. Okay? So that changes the whole ground, the whole playing field, and how you're going to treat the disease. Because if it's a metabolic disease, why are you irradiating people? They say "Because I got to stop the tumor growth!" But if we can stop it by taking away the fuels then we don't need to do that.

Now, of course you are relabeling what the disease is. And by relabeling and providing the evidence that this is a different disease than what we thought... and that the gene mutations are really red herrings, they're epiphenomena! They're very little related to what goes on.

Well, that's a different difficult pill to swallow. After spending hundreds of millions of dollars on the cancer genome project (you might as well flushed it all down). Just to emphasize still how bad it is:

During Obama's administration they had what they called the "moonshot", 100 million dollars given to cancer research... remember the moonshot? Joe Biden was gonna take charge of this, I don't know if he's still doing it. But the moonshot was to... all in immunotherapies. Right?

So I said to people "Take the money, put it into a rocket capsule and send it to the moon! It's not going to help anybody on this planet!" The whole absurdity is that we keep throwing money at a problem, for a disease that we never had. It's not a genetic disease! So we just perpetuate, the 1,600 people keep going up and up and up because we're treating it as if it were genetic... it's not a genetic disease.

The paradigm change has to be:
1. It's not a genetic disease
2. It's a mitochondrial metabolic disease
3. The treatments that you use can be totally different than the ones we're using right now

And if people want to live...

The other problem is we've separated the cancer into several different tribes: Breast cancer tribe is different from lung cancer tribe, brain cancer, colon cancer, all the different cancers. They all think everybody has a different genetic disease. It's all the same!

Once the tribes get together and become united and march on Washington... just like the Million Man March and the Women March and these kind of marches, we have to get the Cancer March. Believe me, it'll happen real quick, you know. It'll happen real quick.

You got all these politicians that are all bought off by the pharmaceutical industry. They're gonna have to say "Hey, listen, they're gonna burn my house down if I don't do something quick!"

Foucher:
Right. And everyone has someone in their life who's been affected by it.

Dr. Seyfried:

Yeah, Well, I think what that does is: You get an outrage on the part of the survivors. Or the people that even have the disease. There's an outrage, an anger that's unquenchable.

Because if you look at your loved ones who have passed away and suffered as horrificly as they have and then you realize they never needed to do that in the first place and you're sitting there thinking "What the hell happened here?" There has to be some outrage! And the outrage is going to motivate the population to do something!

But if the population is complicit with suffering and being treated for a disease they don't have, then there's nothing anybody could about that. Then we're just saying "Okay, whatever." Just like a bunch of sheep, "We'll just take it, we're gonna just have to toughen up, be poisoned, irradiated." Even though we know we don't have that kind of a disease!

We have an epidemic of cancer all over the world, perpetuated by a misunderstanding of what the nature of the disease is. And it has built an infrastructure of massive financial dominance to keep the status quo on that disease. And the people are just being fed misinformation on television, all this kind of stuff.

So it's a big problem. It's really big and if CrossFit can make a dent in this, my hats off to them.

Foucher:

Well, thank you! I was just gonna say thank you for shedding light on this and for writing your book and for doing the due diligence to bring this information to more people. It's because of that that CrossFit can use their platform to then try to spread it to more people. And help to bring the information out there.

Dr. Seyfried:

I think that CrossFit is morphing into something different than what it might have been at the very beginning. You know, at first it was just keeping people physically fit.

Now it seems to be striking at the very heart of chronic diseases. With a philosophy that goes not only for the diet or for the exercise... but now, it's even branching out into recognizing alternative approaches that might even be better. And therefore, they could be a big voice and hitting far more people than a paper written in *Science* or *Nature* or *Cell*, that only a handful of people on the planet can actually read.

88

Foucher:

Right! And we're seeing this over and over again, we've talked about it this week, the solutions coming from the bottom-up rather than top-down and from the patients and the people bringing those solutions and taking their health into their own hands. So it's an exciting time.

Dr. Seyfried:

I think it is! There's light at the end of the tunnel!

Foucher:

It definitely is. Alright, I want to finish with three quick questions I ask everyone on the podcast. The first one is: Three things that you do on a regular basis that have the biggest positive impact on your health?

Dr. Seyfried:

Okay. So... I skip breakfast on probably four days a week.

Foucher:

Okay. Usually weekdays, or...?

Dr. Seyfried:

Weekdays, yeah. I do that and then I work out 4 or 5 times a week at the gym.(...)

So if you try to get a fast in, fast as long as you can. If you can get an 18 hour fast, 4 days a week, that's good. And then what I usually do is eat a handful of nuts, like walnuts, almonds, pecans and maybe a cashew or something - and then I don't eat until dinner.

But then I do eat carbs... which I probably shouldn't do. But I tell you, it's just so good!

Foucher:

Yeah, it's so delicious!

Dr. Seyfried:

They're so delicious! You know, rice, I eat rice. I eat potatoes. But we're trying to reduce it more. My wife is more rigid about it than I am. But, I mean, I drink beer. I drink wine, I drink whiskey. It's not like...

Foucher:

You enjoy your life.

Dr. Seyfried:

Yeah! I mean, you try to keep it in moderation as best as you can. But you also have exercise and fasting as part of the routine. So if I were ever to get cancer, I would be doing a much more aggressive metabolic therapy than I presently do.

There are always some zealots that want to abolish every kind of a risk factor in their life. They won't eat any anything that doesn't produce ketones, you know. Or they insist on exercising all the time. But I'm not that kind of a guy. I don't do that stuff. I go to a bar and drink beer! But not all the time.

Foucher:
I like that approach. You weigh your risks and benefits, you look at where you are at this moment and what makes most sense for you and your lifestyle. And it's true, what's right for you may be very different from what's right for someone else or someone who has cancer.

Dr. Seyfried:
You're right and if I were to have cancer I would be more rigid in maintaining my metabolic management. I'm not doing it now, but... I mean, I do enough. I do it but not to the extent you would do it if you were to try to kill tumor cells.

But yeah, I should be doing it more. I know what to do if I had to do it, let's put it that way.

Foucher:
You're informed.

Dr. Seyfried:
I know where the life preservers are!

Foucher:
There you go! Well, that maybe answers my next question. My next one is: What's one thing that you think would have a big impact on your health but you have a hard time implementing it?

Dr. Seyfried:
Well, I think getting rid of all carbs. Not all but I would say, the starchy carbs. And... it's not easy. You're living in a world of temptations. You go out to dinner with people, they put bread on the table. You can't take the waiter and beat them over the head and say "I don't want the bread!" There's always somebody on the table who wants the bread.

Foucher:
We're constantly surrounded by it. That's hard.

Dr. Seyfried:
Yes, it's hard! You do the best you can. But you know what you have to do if you're informed, at least you have the knowledge base to say "If I do this, I'm going to be better!" Without any information you don't know what to do and put yourself at more risk.

Foucher:
Right. The worst situation is seeing or talking to patients who still have no understanding of what would be a healthy way for them to eat or a way to cure their diabetes if they wanted to. At least if you present that information to people then they can make an informed choice.

Dr. Seyfried:
Absolutely, absolutely.

Foucher:
Last question is: What does a healthy life look like to you ?

Dr. Seyfried:
Well, I can't say what I do is the healthiest. But I can say that it's not the worst. You know, I don't eat pizza every day. In fact, after we heard about the pizza thing at that talk, I said "God damn!" I love pizza, you know! Who doesn't like pizza? (...)
Everybody loves pizza, right? But eating a piece of pizza now puts you at risk for... it takes two weeks to get rid of the damage that a pizza does?

Foucher:
Right, that's what we learned this morning. That changes that whole 'cheat night' mentality a little bit, makes you think about it a little bit more.

Dr. Seyfried:
There's a certain thing... through being happy with your life and not overdoing certain things. But humans are an addictive species. We overdo a lot of things, we exceed in what we're supposed to do.

Foucher:
Especially CrossFit humans. We have a tendency to overdo things.

Dr. Seyfried:
Yes! I mean you guys are nuts with this stuff! But it works, right? But the the so-called 'completely moderate person' is a rare person to be

found, you know. Like my wife, in some ways. She has two wines every night. Never one, never three. It's always two.

Foucher:
She's consistent.

Dr. Seyfried:
Consistent in this moderate behavior. Where I might have three wines or no wine.

Foucher:
Right. The average is still the same.

Dr. Seyfried:
Yeah, but it comes in bursts into rather than... you try to do the best you can. And being aware of this and that's pretty much it. So we'll just keep plowing ahead, find out how long we can survive on the planet.(...)

You know, if you're healthy and engaged, then life is not bad. But if you're depressed and miserable and in pain and... You know, a lot of people commit suicide. They can't handle it. They can't handle life for whatever reason.

A lot of it is metabolic imbalances. Their worldview is just so bleak and so morbid and that shouldn't be! If you're in metabolic homeostasis there is no reason to have these feelings that you need to commit suicide!

That's a big thing, you know. We have a lot of people committing suicide. And you can see post-traumatic stress disorder and all this kind of stuff, that all impacts you. We can understand that, but it also screwed up your metabolism some fierce.

You're on the wrong diet, you're on the wrong lifestyle, your sleep cycle, everything is screwed up. Life is not fun. We all go through tragedies. You have deaths in the family, accidents, you know. You have all kinds of things, job loss, marriage dissolving, you have all these kinds of things.

But if you're metabolically balanced, a lot of times you can handle it. We can do that. It's the people that are completely out of metabolic balance that this becomes too crushing for them and they just can't handle it.

So maintaining the metabolic balance can allow you to survive life.

Foucher:
It's so true.(...)

You don't have to fall so far if you're in peak physical and biochemical condition.

Dr. Seyfried:
Yeah. And it's still hard. I mean, if you have kids and one of your kids gets sick, everything in your life just changes. You get off your schedules and all kinds of things.

But the other thing, too, one last thing is:

To do the kind of research that we do, it's not easy to get funding for this. And we want to thank CrossFit for their support of this work and Travis Christofferson's foundation.

So people who want to make contributions to this kind of work, they can support Travis's foundation. It's called the **Foundation For Metabolic Cancer Therapies.**

It used to be called *Single Cause Single Cure.* Because that's where the support comes from. Because the NIH, they're all locked into the gene theory so most of that money goes to hunt down mutations. Not all of it but a lot of it does.
But in any event that's the way we keep going.

Foucher:
Absolutely! We'll link that up so people can find that link if they're interested in contributing.

Dr. Seyfried:
Yeah, thanks. Thanks a lot.

Dr. Seyfried:
Thank you so much for joining me and thank you for all the work you do!

Foucher:
Thanks Julie, it was really nice. I hope it works and we might help somebody!

Chapter 4: The hard facts about cancer and diet. With Dr. Anthony Chaffee

Hello everyone! Today's interview will be with Professor Thomas Seyfried, in what I think is probably the most important interview I've ever done.

Professor Seyfried is one of the world's foremost experts incancer, cancer biology and research. He has actually shown, quite conclusively, that our understanding of cancer is all wrong.

And by being all wrong, our approaches to treating it are all wrong - and so we're not getting the results that we should and could be. So please, if you are a cancer patient or you know anyone with cancer, tell him or her about the information provided in the following conversation.

Dr. Chaffee:

I'm here today with a very special guest, someone whose work I've long admired: Professor Thomas Seyfried of Boston College. Professor Seyfried, thank you so much for joining us! How are you?

Prof. Seyfried:

Thank you very much Anthony, it's a real pleasure to be here! I'm fine.

Dr. Chaffee:

Thanks! For people that aren't familiar with your work, can you tell us a bit about yourself? What you do and some of your current projects.

Prof. Seyfried:

Well, I'm a Professor of biology at Boston College. I teach cancer metabolism, every semester, to a select group of undergraduate and graduate students.

I also teach general biology to the folks that are not science majors. Like the economists, the political science folks and the english majors. To try to increase scientific literacy among the population.

We have a very active research program, supported by private foundations. Our goal is to develop diet / drug therapies for managing cancer. All types of cancer.

So that's our big thrust right now: What are the most efficacious diet / drug combinations that can manage cancer, without inducing toxicity to any of the normal cells or tissues of our body.

What we do then, is:

We collaborate with clinics that are treating cancer patients throughout the world. And we share the knowledge that we have from our pre-clinical studies with the directors of these clinics, so that they can start applying metabolic therapy - non-toxic metabolic therapy - to their patients in these clinics.

And the success that we're hearing coming back is quite astonishing! This is working!

We ferret out everything before we put it on patients, and my clinical colleagues will then apply it to the patient. So we have everything planned in advance and we get forward-feedback information.

What we do is:

We tweak our systems in-house here, to see if we can improve therapeutic efficacy, and then share that again with the clinical groups. And we're constantly making more and more advances and perfections in the strategy - that will eventually become the standard of care for all cancer patients.

That is: **Metabolic therapy.**

Dr. Chaffee:

I certainly hope so! I've read some of your papers, specifically on glioblastoma multiforme. I'm in neurosurgical residency at the moment, so that's obviously the most common thing that we see.

It's an absolutely devastating disease. Obviously, without any sort of treatment, on average people live about 3 months. With treatment, they make it 15 to 18 months. This is a very devastating illness to watch someone have to go through.

You obviously have copious amounts of publications... some of your publications talk about cancer as a metabolic disease. Specifically, as a dysfunction of the mitochondria. Can you talk a bit about that?

Prof. Seyfried:

Yes, this goes back to the work of Otto Warburg in the 1920s, 30s and 40s, where he defined that cancer originated from damage to mitochondria - and that then elicits a whole series of changes: Forcing the cell into a fermentation mechanism to survive.

We have validated and confirmed Warburg's original finding. In order to do that, I went through the scientific literature, looking at electron micrographs, high magnification of mitochondria and tissues...

Because you can't see them under light microscopy. In order to look at the structure of the mitochondria in the cytoplasm of the cell, you really need electron microscopy.

And I looked at all the major cancers, probably representing 95% of all cancer deaths are caused by these kinds of cancers. I went back through the 1950s, 60s, 70s...

Because back then, in a lot of medical schools, people would be looking at cancer tissue with electron microscopy. Then you go to those papers and you look what they found with respect to the number and structure of the mitochondria in those cancer tissues - and invariably, they were abnormal, structurally.

Even if one were to isolate them and look at the biochemistry, it was abnormal. *So we have never found normal mitochondria in any kind of a major cancer!*

If you don't have normal mitochondria, that means your cells are not going to be able to generate energy through normal respiratory systems, like oxidative phosphorylation [Ox-Phos].

And this is exactly what Warburg said! He said mitochondria, oxidative phosphorylation, becomes irreversibly damaged in all cancers, regardless of where they come from. Thereby forcing them into a fermentation mechanism. And that's what the characteristics of all cancer cells are: They ferment!

Warburg knew glucose was... the lactic acid fermentation, derived from glucose, was the major fuel at that time. We have now defined glutamine as a second fermentable fuel.

The field thought for many years that glutamine was being respired. No, it's not respired, it's fermented. So the two fermentation pathways that drive the majority of cancers are a sugar fermentation and an amino acid fermentation. Without the glucose and glutamine, no cancer cell can survive!

So our goal is to scientifically validate this fermentation mechanism for glutamine and show how Warburg was right in his original description - but he also did not have new information which would clarify and resolve this entire cancer issue back then.

And we're in the process of doing this right now.

96

Dr. Chaffee:
Yeah, that's fantastic! So what are some of the things that can disrupt the mitochondria, to make them precipitate cancer. How does that go about?

How does this actually precipitate the genetic mutations, that we see and attribute blame to as causative - but you're saying that that's actually a knock-on effect.

Prof. Seyfried:
Yeah, the mutations are all downstream epiphenomena. As are most symptoms of what people are studying today, they are all downstream:

The angiogenesis, the failure in apoptosis, all these kinds of things. They're all downstream of the original damage to the mitochondria.

So to answer specifically your question: It's called the oncogenic paradox. And this paradox has perplexed the cancer field for decades!

In other words: How is it possible that you could get cancer from a whole range of different kind of insults? What is the common pathophysiological mechanism that could underlie this range of cancer initiators?

For example, some women may get breast cancer from a clogged milk duct, another one may get it from some sort of viral infection. Another one may get it from a unhealed wound.

There's a whole variety of different ways that couldt elicit breast cancer.

You can consider the same thing for colon cancers, bladder cancers, lung cancers or any other kind of cancers.

Of course, smoking would damage the mitochondria in lung tissues and possibly other tissues.

- Intermittent hypoxia
- Radiation
- Chronic inflammation

Any of these kinds of insults could damage the mitochondria of a cell in a particular tissue, leading to dysregulated cell growth in that tissue.

And the definition of cancer is cell division out of control, or dysregulated cell growth. How does that happen?

97

It happens from damage to the mitochondria in populations of cells, in a particular tissue - eliciting a dysregulated growth. And that's the oncogenic paradox.

So you don't always get cancer from a single insult, it could come from a variety of insults. The bottom line is that you end up with cells that are dysregulated in their cell growth - all of which are fermenting.

And it's important to recognize that the mitochondrion of our cells is the controller of the cell cycle! So when that organelle becomes defective, the cell falls back into a a dysregulated cycle.

This is the way all cells on the planet evolved before oxygen came into the atmosphere, 2.5 billion years ago. We had living cells on the planet before oxygen was in the atmosphere. And: They were all fermenting and they all had dysregulated cell growth.

So the cancer cells are simply falling back on these ancient pathways that have always existed, even before respiration... even before the origination of the mitochondria! So the cells are just simply falling back.

And as long as they have fermentable fuels in the environment, they're very difficult to kill. Radiation and chemo and all these things that we use, are not at the heart of the problem.

As a matter of fact, some of the standards of care actually facilitate the availability of fermentable fuels, making the management of the disease impossible!

That's why the current standard of care makes no sense, when one considers the origin of the disease in the concepts of evolutionary biology.

Dr. Chaffee:

I did read a study a number of years ago, where it spoke about people going on a ketogenic diet. Speaking specifically about using ketosis, about mitochondria specifically.

Showing that when in a state of ketosis, your mitochondria were more efficient - and they also increased in number! Is this some sort of mechanism that would protect from cancer?

What is it about eating carbohydrates and not being in ketosis, that just jams up our mitochondria so much?

Prof. Seyfried:

Well, I don't think the carbohydrates jam up the mitochondria. What happens is that excessive amounts of carbohydrates cause an inflammatory condition in the body.

And it's this elevated inflammation, the state of an inflammation, that contributes to the damage.

Sugar itself is not a carcinogen. However: Chronic excessive consumption of carbohydrates can put the body in an imbalanced nutritional state - and that's what elicits the disease.

It's not only cancer, it's
- Type 2 diabetes
- Alzheimer's disease
- Cardiovascular disease

It's essentially: All of the major chronic diseases that we are currently suffering from are the result of excessive amounts of carbohydrates in the diet.

We as a species did not evolve to eat large amounts of carbohydrates. It was only a seasonal kind of situation. A ripe fruit, a ripe berry or something like this would be so sweet. Maybe honey.

It wasn't chronic exposure to high levels of carbohydrates, that are coming from the foods that we presently have in our societies. And that is ultimately the origin of the majority of chronic diseases that we have:

A diet that is does not fit our evolutionary past.

Dr. Chaffee:
Yeah, I would 100% agree with you on that. And that's something that I've argued for a while now.

Which is that the chronic diseases that we're treating nowadays - exactly as you've outlined - are not diseases per se, but toxicities and malnutrition. A toxic buildup of a species inappropriate diet and a lack of species specific nutrition.

Prof. Seyfried:
Yeah.

Dr. Chaffee:
You build up these toxins, as I mentioned to you before this interview.

I got into this when I took cancer biology, we talked about carcinogens at the time, this was 20 years ago... and we were told that there's 136 known carcinogens just in brussels sprouts, and over 100 in mushrooms, and so on.

So plants are obviously using defense chemicals to stop predation or deter predation. These can build up and cause toxic effects on our body.

Prof. Seyfried:
Well, I think that's true for the industrially produced vegetables. I think organic vegetables, using appropriate natural fertilizers, are safe to eat.

The problem is that organic foods are hard to come by. It's not known whether they're really organic or not. I don't think there's any regulatory commission of free-range animals or organic plants.

I mean, this is what we evolved to eat: They were all organic, 50,000 years ago. There was no industrial harvesting of foods.

But I think that organically grown vegetables, with natural fertilizers, I think those would be very healthy. Along with any other free range meat products or things like this.

The problem is: They're not convenient for the majority of people in the society. Driving up to McDonald's, getting a hamburger is a hell of a lot easier than going out and shooting a deer in the woods!

Dr. Chaffee:
Yeah.

Prof. Seyfried:
You know, it's just the way our society is. Our demands on our time and what we do prevent us from actually rebalancing our physiology. But yet, we put ourselves at risk for cancer and all these other chronic diseases by the convenience of our lifestyle.

Dr. Chaffee:
I certainly agree that with any sort of a whole foods approach, you're going to be in much better stead.

One of the things that I wanted to mention is this data from a guy from Berkeley, Professor Bruce Ames. He published in 1989 some work, looking at an comparison of Alar, which was a pesticide used on apples at the time... they were trying to ban it.

He actually showed - looking specifically in mushrooms - that mushrooms had around 10,000 times the amount of natural insecticides and pesticides by weight as the Alar would get sprayed on these plants. And that this amount of plant carcinogens was thus way more likely to cause cancer than the pesticide ones.

But to your point: I agree 100%, obviously pesticides and insecticides, these are toxic by design. They're trying to to kill insects from eating them. So certainly, that's going to make things a lot worse.

Prof. Seyfried:

Well, in my book I showed that a lot of these so carcinogens that you just mentioned *[He is talking about the Alar carcinoges]*, they're taken up in mammalian cells and they actually cause the mitochondria to fluoresce. Biofluorescence.

So those carcinogens are going right to the mitochondria, damaging the mitochondria. Which is then the first step...

The first step in the initiation of cancer is to disrupt oxidative phosphorylation, OxPhos. And only cells that can upregulate a fermentation mechanism as the result of this damage, only those cells can become cancer cells!

Cells that can not upregulate fermentation rarely if ever become tumorogenic. Cells of cardiomyocytes, they can't switch from OxPhos to fermentation. Neurons in the brain rarely become tumorogenic. It's the glial cells, not the neuron. Neurons can't ferment for very long.

So only cells that have the capacity to replace respiration with fermentation can become cancer cells.

Dr. Chaffee:

That's very interesting! And I think that's a good illustration of what the actual mechanism is.

Prof. Seyfried:

Yeah. I mean, it becomes very clear once you understand the biology of the problem. Understanding how we get it and, and more importantly, understanding how we manage it. That becomes very logical.

The problem is: This information is not known by the majority of oncologists or scientists in the field.

Dr. Chaffee:

Absolutely. In addition to that, with my sort of endeavors into nutrition and how this affects disease: Even just the idea that diabetes and heart disease are caused by eating a lot of carbohydrates and sugar, a lot of people really don't know it.

Doctors don't know about these things, nutritionists as well. They still are on the same "Cholesterol will kill you-" idea. Which I think has been thoroughly debunked.

Prof. Seyfried:
Well, it's been debunked - but everybody's popping the statin tablets! Obviously, they still think cholesterol has a big big role in cardiovascular disease. Triglycerides.

You're absolutely right. And in the cancer wards, they still give the cancer patients sugar, coke and ice cream, cake... and they say glucose has nothing to do with cancer.

There's such a lack of knowledge, it's profound, it's unbelievable! The lack of knowledge on the part of the healthcare industry, as to what should and should not be done to keep people healthy.

Dr. Chaffee:
Yeah that's one of the things, I was a bit upset there...

Because I see this every day in the hospital. You know, I see the food that they feed them. It's just sugary carbs, that's it. There's almost no meat, there's certainly no fat. There's a bit of dairy... but it's it's always like chocolate milk, as opposed to just normal milk. Just garbage.

I'm going around seeing our brain tumor patients who just underwent surgery... and here they are, eating all this sugary nonsense.

And I just can't help but think "This is what gave you this problem in the first place - and we're just shoveling it into your face!"

Prof. Seyfried:
Yeah, it drives the tumor. What we also found:

I published a major paper on this, with the standard of care for brain cancer: The very treatments that are used, the radiation, as well as Temazolamide, they free up massive amounts of glucose and glutamine in the tumor micro environment - making long-term survival very, very rare!

So it's the therapies themselves that... In other words, it's bad enough to have a glioblastoma - it's even worse to use standard of care to treat it! Because you've more or less signed and sealed the death certificate of this patient.

The human brain should rarely - if ever - be irradiated. This is nonsense, this has to stop!

I published a clear paper on how the radiation breaks apart the glutamine- glutamate cycle in the brain, freeing up massive amounts of glutamine. And the steroids they give these patients increase blood sugar.

So the two fuels necessary causing cancer cells to grow out of control are made available, in abundant quantities, by the very treatments that we're doing to these patients.

Dr. Chaffee:
Yeah...

Prof. Seyfried:
We have made no advance in glioblastoma therapy in almost 100 years. My most recent paper shows, in 100 years...

We have a telescope that now orbits 1 million miles from earth to look at the very origins of our solar system - we do that, and yet we've made no advance in glioblastoma!

And many other cancers. Once you have metastatic lung cancer, a colon cancer, the survival is so much less. Because the treatments we're using contribute to the demise of these patients. It's unbelievable!

Dr. Chaffee:
Yeah, absolutely.

Prof. Seyfried:
A tragedy, it's actually a tragedy.

Dr. Chaffee:
Right, and chemo can be so hard on people. I don't know what people are more concerned with: Like getting cancer - or getting cancer and realizing that means they need chemo. Because I've had friends, and obviously patients, devastated by by these treatments.

Prof. Seyfried:
Yeah, I think they fear the treatment as much as they do the disease. They think their hair is going to fall out, they're going to bleed from the gums, they're going to be sick and tired all the time. Some people recover really well.

Actually, there are some reports now that show water-only therapeutic fasting can significantly reduce some of the toxic effects of chemotherapy.

But my point is: Why would you want to use chemotherapy, when we know we just have to pull the plug on the fermentable fuels? With diet and drugs that aren't so toxic? Especially when under therapeutic ketosis.

I mean, there's a clear framework and strategy for managing cancer without toxicity. The biggest problem is there is no business model to support this. Which is the singular greatest inhibitor of moving this forward.

People haven't found out how to make money on metabolic therapy. Yet! That's the biggest problem. It's not the patient that should be benefited, it's how to make revenue from this.

I think the entrepreneur will come, and the entrepreneur will figure out how to do this. I'm not that kind of a person. My job is: How do we keep cancer patients alive with a higher quality of life, beyond what they were ever predicted to to have.

Dr. Chaffee:
Yeah. I suppose a good business model would be just setting up clinics, that have this treatment regime and actually get results - and then people will go to them.

Prof. Seyfried:
We're doing that now, actually. We have some clinics...

But some of the drugs that we use like a 6-Diazo-5-oxo-L-norleucine (DON) is not available to the public. And it really bothers me, because that was used on children and cancer patients and patients with other indications in the past.

But yet, if you try to get it, the drug administration would say "It's not for human use, not for human consumption." That should not be, because that drug is very powerful, especially when used in ketosis.

We did the experiments. We showed the results... and hundreds and hundreds of cancer patients are emailing me "How do I get this drug?"

The answer is "Write your senator or congressman! They should make this legal to get!" Because it's a drug that has to be repurposed.

It was used on cancer, but it wasn't used in the right way. If you don't know how to use the tool, it's not going to give you the outcome that you would expect.

They say "Oh, it's too toxic" - relative to what? Chemo and radiation? No, not even close!

So we have a drug available right now, that can be used to reduce cancer in so many patients - when used with nutritional therapeutic ketosis. We've already shown how it works, and it works really well. And it should be used right now! But it's not, because there's no profit in this drug.

So when there's no profit, we can't use it, regardless of the patient. Can you believe this is? This is what we call a moral issue.

Dr. Chaffee:
Is there any way to sort of push through, getting it approved by the FDA? To get this going? Or is it there's just no money...

Prof. Seyfried:
You know, I think it's all revenue generation. I'm sorry to say that. The FDA will approve drugs if there's a proof of concept. Nothing could be stronger than the proof of concept of how this drug DON works with ketosis. Nothing is as strong as this!

Yet, it won't be approved - because there's no revenue to be generated from this.

It's a business model! People have to realize that is a revenue generating disease. Hospitals use drugs and radiation because they generate so much revenue from the insurance companies.

So are we interested in keeping people alive longer? Yes! But it seems only, if it can be associated with revenue generation.

If it's not associated with revenue generation, I'm sorry: We have to sacrifice those cancer patients. There it is.

Dr. Chaffee:
Yeah. I'm in Australia at the moment, so a there's a public and a private health care system here. But regarding the public system:

Obviously, this is coming from the government. And there are massive delays within this system, so it can actually take 4.5 years for someone to get into our clinic.

With like radiculopathy, a compressed nerve in their spine, that needs surgery. 4 and a half years is our current wait list for that. So there are a lot of delays and there are a lot of issues.

But we deal with a lot of cancer as well, those get obviously treated right away because it's a life or death emergency. But the government really tries hard to not pay for anything that gets done, and they put a lot of roadblocks in the way.

And I just wonder: Wouldn't this be something that would be attractive to them? Because this is eminently more cheaper than the actual standard treatments. I think that... Well, you may have some ideas?

Maybe it's that a lot of hospitals and systems around the world that have a public model, generally try to emulate the guidelines set in America in the private system with the insurance, sort of driving things.

Prof. Seyfried:

Yeah, you would think so. You would think this would be the best thing for governments to cut their medical bills. No. No, no. There's a force, there's a power that's controlling this. Even though the governments would like to do it.

The IRB, institutional review boards, have shut down this so many times. They want to do standard of care first, before they do metabolic therapy. Why?

Well, there's something else going on here. And again, it has to do with the control of the entire medical system. What we call standard of care.

Care standard of care should have never been written in granite.

But it seems to have been written in granite.

In other words: You can use metabolic therapy only after you demonstrate that conventional chemo and radiation don't work. Now, for glioblastoma, 99% of the time they don't work!

So why do we have to continue to push ineffective therapies? And once we realize they don't work, then we maybe want to do metabolic therapy?

No, no, no. You should do metabolic therapy first! That's the number one. Do metabolic therapy first, and then you'll be shocked at how you won't need toxic radiation and chemicals.

And that is not what the system wants to hear. Period.

Dr. Chaffee:

Well, that obviously needs to change somehow. I don't know...

Prof. Seyfried:

Yes, but who's going to change it?

Dr. Chaffee:

Right, I don't know.

Prof. Seyfried:

The bottom line is: You just keep treating patients with metabolic therapy and let the patients be the advocates of what's going on. Let them go out and tell people what they did. "Why are you still alive? How come you're not dead? You should have been dead three years ago, and you're out here working in your garden!"

He'll tell you. Those guys will be more than happy to tell you what they did.

Dr. Chaffee:
Well, that's the thing... not even to the extent that you're talking about, actual treatment modalities with diet and drugs.

I had a friend of mine who was diagnosed with glioblastoma multiforme, about 6 years ago. And I had already been involved in this sort of research, seeing a lot work from yourself and others.

I just said "Hey look, there's a lot of evidence here that suggests that at least being on a ketogenic diet is going to be very beneficial" - I sort of pitched a carnivore diet because that's my thing.

But she didn't do a whole carnivore diet, diet she did more keto. But she had a lot more meat. She cut out the carbs, she stopped drinking... and she's now 6 years still alive! At 5 years, she had an MRI - and she had no sign of disease!

Unfortunately, it did come back in her sixth year. So she's sort of undergoing a further debulking. But 5 years and her 5-year MRI was clear. That's almost unheard of with GBM.

Prof. Seyfried:
Well, see: Those kinds of cases need to need to be written up. The patient that we wrote up, Pablo Kelly, who has a website and talks about his survival:

He chose no standard of care, just metabolic therapy. And he was on a carnivore kind of diet.

So he's out now 8 years. And his tumor is not gone, it's there. He has a debulking surgery every three years. No radiation or chemo.

I'll give you the full story, a very kind of a colorful guy from Devon, England. He used the carnivore procedure. No carbs, he cut all that stuff out. And he's still going fine, he's had two children.

He was 26 when he was diagnosed, lived a 'horrible lifestyle', as he said. Alcohol, drugs and bad food, all that kind of stuff. Of course, after his tumor diagnosis, he became very pristine in what he was doing - and he's still doing fine!

There's two things we think need to happen.

1) Avoiding the standard of care
2) Switching your entire diet lifestyle over to zero or very low carbohydrate

Whether you do that with carnivore or whether you do it with plants... you can you can do it with either or.

We developed the glucose-ketone index calculator (GKI), to allow people to know whether or not they're in a state of nutritional ketosis by blood markers. You can do Keto-Mojo, that's a blood glucose-ketone meter.

So the cancer patient knows what is going on metabolically. And when Pablo went off his diet a little bit, the tumor started to grow again - and you could see it on MRI! And immediately, he threw himself back into a very low GKI index. Then, you could see the tumor stopped growing. It was very clear.

Cancer cells can't burn ketones or fats, they only can burn glucose and glutamine. But there's no diet that will target glutamine.

So patients always ask "Oh, what am I going to eat to target glutamine?" Glutamine is the most abundant amino acid in our body, it's not gonna work with any kind of diet I'm afraid.

Now, I'm shocked at how long people can live with just ketogenic diets or these kinds of things. But if we ever married those diets with the glutamine targeting drug DON, I think we could eliminate these tumors in the majority of people very quickly!

We're not doing that. We're not doing the very things we need to do to make cancer a very manageable disease, without suffering great toxicity.

Why are we not doing this? Because
- Nobody knows about it, they simply don't know it. And
- The ones that are in charge don't want to believe it

If you go to most of the oncology centers, they say "There's no evidence to support metabolic therapy. If it were so important and effective, we would all know about it"

Wrong! You wouldn't know about it. You're dealing with huge profits for an entire industry here, let's be honest. Right?
Dr. Chaffee:

Absolutely, yeah. So with the DON, going to the drug and diet cocktail: Obviously, they're not letting us use this in humans. But you've done quite extensive animal models and experiments, is that right?

Prof. Seyfried:

Yes. We've looked at it in a variety of metastatic and invasive brain cancers and things like this. I mean, all of these drugs... DON was used in humans! It was used in little kids with leukemia.

So it's not like it's a drug that's never been used in humans. Of course it's been used. It's in malaria treatments, there's a lot of ways that that drug has already been used. But not for cancer.

Of course, don't you think the pharmaceutical industry knows about glutamine targeting? Sure they do!

So what they do is: They build drugs that are not nearly as effective as DON, patent that drug and then throw that drug out on the cancer population, but never using keto with it.

You get some therapeutic benefit, maybe. But you're not going to get the full therapeutic benefit.

Cancer can be managed with drug / diet cocktails. People need to know that!

We clearly showed how nutritional ketosis can facilitate the delivery of these drugs to tumor cells, three times more. That means you can lower the doses, reduce the toxicity and increase the efficacy of the whole process.

We know the framework, we know how to manage cancer. Without toxicity. The problem is: It won't be used in the clinics - for a variety of different reasons.

The people themselves have to rise up and say "I want metabolic therapy!"Forget about all this crazy nuking and poisoning people. I mean, it's not based on we understand the biology of the disease to be.

So who's going to make the change? The guys at the top medical schools? No. It's going to be the people themselves.

Who will benefit most from metabolic therapy? The cancer patients will benefit most from metabolic therapy. They need to understand this, they need to rally, they need to do something. Put pressure on your government officials and these kinds of things. Then it will happen.

It's never going to happen when you're trying to convince Big Pharmacy and big medical schools that metabolic therapy is the way to go. Because it's not going to generate the replacement revenue. So you have to have something that's going to give replacement revenue.

In my mind, I want to see how many people can survive long term. Like your friend, like Pablo Kelly. Like many others who should have been dead a long time ago. People who are living a hell of a lot longer with a higher quality of life.

What's wrong with that? Why is this being resistant? Why is there resistance against this? Makes no sense to me.

Dr. Chaffee:

Yeah, especially with something like cancer. If there was ever something to rally behind, I think cancer is it. Anyone you talk to around the world, they always have sympathy for cancer and people that get it.

So I'm just amazed that these things aren't...

Prof. Seyfried:

Well, the other thing you have to keep in mind is that the term cure has been a very reactive kind of term. We never use that term, we don't say "A metabolic therapy can cure cancer". What metabolic therapy can do is allow the patient to live longer. It's a management strategy.

You can manage the disease. Okay? In other words, you don't have to die so quickly. You can live a lot longer.

If you have cancer at your age - you look very healthy - suppose you get cancer and you manage it with metabolic therapy. And you die at 99 from a heart attack. Well, you obviously were cured from your cancer, because it didn't kill you.

But we don't know whether anybody is cured using metabolic therapy. All we know is that they seem to live longer than their were predicted with a higher quality of life. What's wrong with that? What is wrong with that scenario?

Dr. Chaffee:

Yes, and not being burned down by like the chemo and radiation!

Prof. Seyfried:

Yeah. I mean, let's be honest: Don't forget, we have millions of cancer survivors who have survived toxic radiation and chemo. But their body pays a significant price for that. They're suffering from

- gastrointestinal problems
- psychiatric problems
- hormonal imbalances
- microbiome disturbances

All kinds of things that make their life less enjoyable, less pleasurable. Because they were exposed to toxic poisons and toxic radiation.

This is stone age treatment, this should not happen in today's day and age. When we understand the biology of the disease very clearly. And yet, we're doing these crazy things to these poor people. It doesn't make any sense to me

Dr. Chaffee:
I had a very good friend of mine that I grew up playing rugby with. And he unfortunately contracted sarcoma in his sinuses. Probably when he was in his late 30s, early 40s. A very fit guy, very active guy.

He went on and off, kept going... he struggled along with this for about three years: One of the chemo agents that he used just completely destroyed his nerves. He became almost crippled from this. Just from basically half a course of this chemotherapy.

And he stopped it! He just said... even though the cancer was was responding well to it. He just said "Look, I don't want to survive cancer to be a cripple and an invalid. I'm not gonna take that anymore."

Prof. Seyfried:
Right. I have hundreds and hundreds of situations like this. Because I have thousands of people emailing me - and they always have a story.

What I feel so bad about is that they always contact me after they've been suffered through the standards of care. And their stories are horrific! I mean, you can't torture human beings as well as what some of the standard of care does to people.

I don't even think waterboarding would be as bad as some of the treatments they give these cancer patients. This is tragic! It's a tragedy of monumental proportions - and we don't have to do this!

Some of the chemotherapies our colleagues in Turkey use what we call a metabolically supported chemotherapy:

They use the lowest doses of chemo together with nutritional ketosis - which has really good outcomes. And they said they would prefer not to use any chemotherapy, but they're forced to do it by the system!

So the system of treatment seems to have permeated all healthcare industries in societies throughout the world. You go to India... I was shocked at how they love radiation over there, they radiate everybody over there. Any kind of a cancer.

I thought various cultures would be more open to metabolic therapy, but there seems to be a lock hold on cancer treatments throughout the world. They have to do this radiation and chemo. Now it's immunotherapy.

The problem with CAR-T immunotherapy... such a costly and very complicated therapy. What are they doing? Why are they doing this?

All they have to do is pull the plug on the glucose and glutamine, while under nutritional ketosis - and you don't have to spend 265,000 dollars to have your cancer managed! You see what I'm saying?

It comes right down to this whole concept of "What is cancer?

Is it a genetic disease? Or is it a mitochondrial metabolic disease?

And once you realize that it's a mitochondrial metabolic disease, most of the treatments we're doing to the cancer patients make no sense. They're not based on the fundamental underlying what the disease is.

So I don't know what I have what we have to do to get the word out. But somebody has to know about this. Otherwise, we're just going to continue to kill these poor patients, year in and year out. Let's be honest.

Dr. Chaffee:
Yeah.

Prof. Seyfried:
I don't know what it is in Australia, in the United States alone, we have over 1,600 people dying every single day from cancer. Over 1,600.

When I was in China, it's 8,000! Because their population is large. As a matter of fact: In China, cancer has replaced heart disease as the number one killer of their population.

Dr. Chaffee:

Jesus!
Prof. Seyfried:
So what the hell is going on here?

And they're always saying "Oh, we're making major breakthroughs!" I ask where's the breakthroughs? With a breakthrough, he death rate should drop!

There's no breakthroughs. It's business as usual. More and more cancer deaths, no accountability.

I tell you, we're always running around, raising money for cancer patients. You know, let's do the 5k run for breast cancer. Let's do this!

What do they do with all the money that you get for raising? They give it to the people who think cancer's a genetic disease, keeping the system in place.

I mean, it's nuts. We got to start wisen up, people have to start asking "Where the hell is the accountability for the money that I'm raising?"

The only people who get healthy are the ones running and swimming to raise money for cancer research. You get healthy doing a bike ride – but with that money you're raising, you poison and irradiate the people that you're raising the money for!

It doesn't make any sense, does it?
Dr. Chaffee:
No, no. And that's the thing too, a good point that you raised: Cancer rates are getting worse. Like cancer eclipsing heart disease in China as the number one killer.

I looked at some of the gross figures in the US. I was looking at the numbers since we sort of overhauled our diet, after the 1977 USDA declaration that cholesterol is going to cause heart disease. And we reduced our fat and cholesterol intake by about 30%, reduced red meat by about 33%.

And we increase fruits and vegetables 30, 40%, increased carbs, increased sugar, all these things.

Since then, there's been roughly an overall tripling in cancer rates in the United States! You know, that cannot be genetic.
Prof. Seyfried:
No, no.
Dr. Chaffee:
Anyone who studies populations genetics knows very well that it's not possible to do that in a limited number of generations.

That means there's something in the environment that has changed and has affected this.

Prof. Seyfried:

Well, here's the other statistic that's often used to say we're making major advances in cancer:

The anti-smoking campaign that started probably around 1990, 1991...

Cancer was associated with smoking, so people stopped smoking. So if you use the 1991 rate of increase compared to today and you say "Look at how much how fewer cancer patients we have today!" - based on 1991 data.

Yeah, because everybody was smoking and dying in 1991! Not everyone, but many people were smoking and dying.

But if you look at the number of dead bodies accumulating every year, the number of dead bodies accumulate at the same percentage as the population growth.

So every year, the number of dead people from cancer goes up. The American Cancer Society has all the numbers, they all publish it every year. So this is a well documented event.

That numbers of dead people increase every year. Still: You don't use a 1991 rate to predict the success in the field!

"Oh, if we had continued to smoke in 2022, we would have had a lot more dead cancer deaths."Of course you would, if people hadn't stopped smoking.

So the only real major advance we made was prevention – by the people. This had nothing to do with the science. We stopped smoking and therefore lung cancer numbers reduced.

And lung cancer is still the number one killer. But it would have killed a hell of a lot more if we hadn't stopped smoking.

But the treatments... you have to look at: Are there any new treatments that reduce cancer deaths? And the answer is nope. Zero! So it's a tragedy, no matter how you look at it.

Yet, the poor people in the hospital are suffering immensely, hair falling out... I say anytime you see a bald cancer patient, that person was treated by someone who doesn't understand the biology of the disease they're working on.

You shouldn't be bald, you're trying to kill cancer cells! What the hell? Why is your hair falling out? "Oh, the hair and the cancer cells share some common features - they're both growing."

114

But you don't want to kill all your good cells! Your gut cells, your hair cells, those have to be killed off? That tells me you have no idea.

Furthermore, they use these terms precision medicine. Well, how in the hell is your hair falling out with this so called precision medicine? Oh, it was "off target". if it's so precise - how come we have all these off-target effects on the person's body? I mean, this is such a bunch of crap.

When are they going to wise up to understand what's going on here. It just doesn't make any sense!

Dr. Chaffee:
Yeah, that's another thing, too. Something that you pointed out.

In a cancer, like a tumor:

In medical school, obviously you get taught these genetic changes, and then this tumor just starts propagating. And all of the tumorcells shouls have the same DNA, monoclonal. But that's not what we see, we don't see that in tumors.

We see certain ones that have certain hallmarks and changes, increased mitosis. But a lot of these things just look normal they. They just look like normal tissue.

And yet, they behave as cancer. That to your point is: If these all have varying genetics, why are they all acting the same? That definitely looks like a downstream effect, as opposed to a causative effect.

Prof. Seyfried:
Oh yeah, absolutely! Absolutely. But everyone of the cells in that tumor is fermenting. They all have different genetic characteristics, but they're all fermenting.

So why are we so concerned about targeting the genetic mutations that differ in every single cell of the body - when the tumor cells are all fermenting?

That's the power of the somatic mutation theory. If the somatic mutation theory says cancer is caused by genetic mutations, mindlessly we go out and try to target all these different genetic mutations.

The mitochondrial metabolic theory says that they're all fermenting. The field has not yet accepted the mitochondrial metabolic theory as the origin of cancer, as Warburg had originally stated. They threw him under the bus.

When Watson and Crick first discovered the DNA structure, everybody ran off like the lemmings over the cliff, chasing DNA mutations. It's like the dog chasing his tail.

Now we've come to realize that all that genomic ideas, millions and billions of dollars spent on all this genomic stuff...

What we're finding, though - which is very interesting now – is that there are certain spontaneous mutations, that actually interfere with glucose and glutamine metabolism.

We call these therapeutic mutations - they're actually god's gift to the cancer patient by a rare event. Nobody knows.

Like Pablo Kelly, he has an IDH1 mutation. It's called IDH1. This IDH1 mutation produces a metabolite called 2-hydroxyglutarate.

We and others have found that 2-hydroxyglutarate interferes with the glutamineolysis pathway, driving the energy of the tumor. And also the glycolysis pathway, building the raw material so the tumor can grow.

So the mutation itself is acting like a drug that can target two of the pathways driving the cancer. Can you believe this?

Dr. Chaffee:

Wow!

Prof. Seyfried:

And people that have this mutation are known to live twice as long as the people who don't have the mutation!

The problem is: Even the people with the mutation are given radiation and chemo, which reduces the ability of the very therapeutic mutation to work, it's unbelievable! *(Laughs)*

So if you don't do standard of care and are fortunate enough to have this therapeutic mutation, you can live a long time.

Pablo has this therapeutic mutation, goes on a carnivore-ketogenic diet. And every three years has had debulking surgery because this indolent tumor just hangs around. But he's never used the DON to target and kill off the rest of it.

So we have a strategy, I think. But it's really...

When you understand the biology of the disease, you can't help but be bewildered and overwhelmed by this new information - and how easy it is to get rid of cancer! Or manage it, let's put it that way. I wouldn't say get rid of it, but certainly manage it. It becomes a clear strategy.

It's just that more and more people need to know about this. And once they know, there'll be a stampede for this.

Dr. Chaffee:

Yeah. What are some of the cancers that you found, that are more susceptible and sensitive to this metabolic treatment?

Prof. Seyfried:

Well, the alternative question is which cancers have I found to be resistant? Okay? This is because almost everyone is susceptible!

Every lung cancer that we've looked at, every breast, colon, bladder, kidney cancer - they're all very prone. They all have to ferment.

All the blood cancers are all driven by glutamin. So you're talking about all the major cancers.

You know, here's the situation: There are reports in the scientific literature, showing a genetically engineered mouse that has a genetically engineered lung cancer - that doesn't respond to metabolic therapy.

Now, the problem is, we don't know any human being walking around the planet, that has been genetically engineered the same way as this mouse has been genetically engineered. Nor does that person have a genetically engineered lung tumor.

Until we can find that person and ask that individual why they're not responding to metabolic therapy, I don't know.

But all of our mouse models that we found, all have naturally arising cancers. In other words: The cancer arose naturally in the natural host.

This is the best model that you can use because it's the same kind of cancer that would be found in dogs, a dog cancer arising naturally in the dog host. A human cancer arising naturally in the human host.

Those are the kinds of cancers that respond to metabolic therapy. Some of these genetically engineered things are not responsive in some ways. What reasons for, I have no clue.

I don't know why a mouse that's been so genetically engineered - with both the host and the cancer - doesn't respond to metabolic therapy. But I think I'll let somebody else figure that one out.

But who cares about that? Who gives a rat's ass about a mouse that's been genetically engineered, that doesn't respond to metabolic therapy? Right? Let's focus our attention on natural cancers.

Like dogs, for example: They respond remarkably well! Dogs with cancer. Cancer kills so many dogs. It's like the number one killer of domestic dogs.

The wolf never has rarely cancer. I don't think there's been a cancer in the literature, it must be very rare, in a wolf. Because they're eating natural, they're eating their natural diet in the wild.

They're not pounding down big burgers or jelly filled donuts, this kind of thing. And then, if you go to the zoo and ask the zookeeper "Why are you feeding your chimpanzees their natural diet? Why are giving them their natural diet? Why don't you let them eat jelly filled donuts and pizza, and drink Coca-Cola?"

What the zookeeper told me down here at the Franklin Park Zoo in Boston "Oh that would be animal cruelty. Animal abuse!" - and I'm saying "What the hell man! We're 98% similar to the chimpanzees, their DNA!" Right?

Let's take chimps and put them on an American diet from the time they're weaned. Let's take 100 chimps from the time they're weaning and give them only what we eat. Not their natural diet.

What do you think is going to happen?

- Cancer
- Dementia
- Type 2 diabetes
- Obesity

All the same sh*t that we have would be seen! But you can't do that because it's animal abuse!

Dr. Chaffee:

Yeah. Well, and that's it. They have the signs, saying "Do not feed the animals! This isn't their natural food!" They get very sick. And then we put that same nonsense into our mouths... and don't think that anything bad is going to happen.

Prof. Seyfried:

No, we get very, very sick! And the food industry and the pharmaceutical industry are both linked.

I had one of my students go and look at the investigation between the two organizations. Like, the big food industries producing all these foods that are poorly nutritious and full of highly processed carbs, that make you sick.

And on the other end of the other spectrum, the pharmaceutical companies will give you drugs and therapies to try to make you healthy.

Dr. Chaffee:
Yeah, exactly.

Prof. Seyfried:
What an industry! Right? It's unbelievable. It drives the economy... so I guess we have to be happy, because many of us are doing well - based on the revenue generation from these two industries overlapping with each other.

But I think that prevention is one thing. People who know about this certainly can...

Even Otto Warburg said you can't get cancer if your mitochondria remain healthy. And that's true, you can't get cancer if your mitochondria are healthy. That's prevention.

But we live in a society where it's hard not to eat. Okay, I saw you cooking the giant tomahawk rib eye. Well, I think that's wonderful and I would eat it - but also with a big baked potato, and a big loaf of bread with butter slathered all over it. And a big pile of unhealthy vegetables.

(Both laughing)

I mean, everybody would go down that path. But eating the tomahawk ribeye by itself... well, I don't know about that. But I certainly would do something like that.

Dr. Chaffee:
Yeah, that's funny... I was gonna say, too...

One of the things I thought, exactly as you said, is that we don't see cancers in wild animals - and we don't see them in the zoo. Everyone says that "Well, animals in the wild, they probably don't live long enough to get cancer." But that never explains animals in the zoo. Or "They're active and they're running around."

But an animal in the zoo is sitting around its whole life - and they don't get these cancers. The cancer rates in dogs and cats, these have all increased dramatically since the inception of packaged dog and cat food.

Prof. Seyfried:

Yeah, yeah, absolutely. And the zoos maintain a very nutritious diet, they have a staff of veterinarians that monitor the diet. They're so carefully monitored, these zoo primates, the gorillas and the chimps, are monitored very carefully. All the time, in regards to nutritional balances.

That's why they said, if we gave them jelly filled donuts and pizza, they would get hammered.

There is a family of chimps that live with humans, they're on the web. It's a group of chimps that live with humans. You should see these chips go wild when they get the jelly sandwiches! They're banging on the table, they're getting all excited eating jelly sandwiches.

Dr. Chaffee:
That's awful!

Prof. Seyfried:
Haha! Yeah, you can go on the web, there's a bunch of chimps that live with a human family. And while they talk, the chimps are pounding down all this stuff. Loving it, banging on the table...

Dr. Chaffee:
...Captain Crunch, just going after it...

Prof. Seyfried:
I mean, who wouldn't? You could drop off your box of donuts into the pen with the chimps down there, they'd be all over the donuts. And the other guys that weren't getting the donuts would be all upset.

It just shows you that we as a species have used technology,,, sweetness in our evolutionary past was only rare and seasonal. But our technology has now made it permanent.

Now we can get this sweet stuff all the time - and we like it! We evolved to like sweets. So everything has been carefully developed, tweaked, to all of our taste buds, to make us want to eat more of this. Even though we put ourselves at risk for cancer, dementia, heart disease, diabetes, all this kind of stuff.

We're willing to still eat the foods that are putting us in that situation, because they taste so good.

Dr. Chaffee:
And to your previous point about this unholy alliance between food and pharmacy:

Dr. Robert Lustig of UCSF, he mentioned in one of his books - if I can remember the numbers correctly – that the sugar industry makes about 1.3 trillion dollars a year, gross figures.

And what we spend just treating the metabolic issues that are derived from sugar consumption is about 2.4 trillion dollars! So this is a massive, massive amount of money. I mean, that's the entire federal budget, just spent on eating and supporting sugar addiction.

Prof. Seyfried:

Yeah, of course. But if a politician came out and said

"Listen, our health health industry budget is crippling our nation. It's actually causing a crisis, putting us at risk. So we're all going to go back and do paleolithic eating! We're going to eat tomahawk rib eyes, we're going to cut down on our carcinogenic vegetables..."

How long do you think that guy's going to remain in office? They'll vote his ass out right away!

But when you have the cancer, then all of a sudden your whole world begins to change, how come I wasn't told about this?!

Well, we're telling you now! Do you want to make the choice or not?

Dr. Chaffee:

So with glioblastoma: In your animal models, what are you finding to be the results when you put them on this, the DON and the restrictive dietary ketosis. How much of a benefit are you seeing in those mice?

Prof. Seyfried:

Oh yeah, we're getting 3, 4 times longer survival.

Dr. Chaffee:

Wow!

Prof. Seyfried:

One of the things we've done... because we took these glioblastoma cells and we identified the metastatic cancer as being a type of plastic macrophage.

And in the GBM, if you look at glioblastoma, many of the so-called mesenchymal cells, the cells that have this mesenchymal phenotype, are the most highly invasive.

They did call it glioblastoma multiforme, because of all the different kinds of cells that you would see in there. The mesenchymal kind of cell is the most invasive.

And when we took those cells out of the brain of the mouse and put them in the flank, they metastasized. They spread all over the body.

Then we found out that all metastatic cancers have macrophage characteristics. So we know the nature of the metastatic cell: It's a type of a macrophage - and it loves glutamine and glucose.

When we put them in the flank, they spread all over the body. We use bioluminescence imaging, we can image the tumor cells and see how much they've spread through the body.

Then... we call them terminal mice. They're going to die in a couple of days. You can see the heavy breathing, you can see their immobility.

Then we hit him with our diet drug cocktail - and within 3 or 4 days, these guys are back, walking around like they never had anything! They still have cancer, but it's been managed.

So: We took these guys from from death's doorstep... normally they would be dead by 30 days if we did nothing. Or if we would just continue to feed them the high carbohydrate standard lab chow.

But then, we got them now to live over 4 and a half months! 5 times longer than they normally would have.

We haven't published this yet, but we plan to publish it. Once we have all the conditions of the drug / diet cocktails defined.

We're seeing it for pediatric cancer in the mice, too. Because we're doing the same thing to these little kids that we do to the adults. We hit them with high-dose chemo, we hit them with high radiation. We do the same toxic things to those little kids as we do to adults.

And we can take these pediatric models that we've developed here at Boston College, and... We can keep these mice alive so much longer and in such a higher quality of life!

We know that we can get the same results in the pediatric clinic as we see with these natural pediatric brain tumors in in the mice. We know we can keep people alive with advanced metastatic cancer, if we do drug diet cocktails at the right time. Don't interfere with this!

Don't forget: With none of our mice, we do radiation [The groups that get meatblic therapy]. So the results that we get...

They say "Oh, you just get all those great results in the mice, you wouldn't see that in the human."

Well, maybe - because we don't irradiate the mice! So if we'd radiate the mice, maybe we'll see what we get in the human. I don't know because we don't plan to do that. And I don't plan to irradiate, why?

Now, I'm not saying radiation is bad for everything. Because I think, if you have a tumor in a particular location, it's well defined, it's not metastatic – then, radiation could potentially cure that kind of a tumor. So we don't want to throw all these things under the bus.

We did temozolomide with metabolic therapy, and we showed that it was no better than... Temozolomide is the primary chemo for brain cancer.

We showed that it was no better than metabolic therapy, used with hyperbaric oxygen.

And the mice never got sick with our metabolic therapy. They got sick with the temozolomide. So we tried Temozolomide with metabolic therapy: We put them all together.

Yeah, they did good, but they didn't do any better than metabolic therapy by itself - without the sickness!

So I'm saying: Why are we doing all this stuff? Why are we doing what we're doing? Because Temozolomide generates huge revenue for the hospital!

Dr. Chaffee:
Yeah.

Prof. Seyfried:
So we're not interested in the revenue generation here, we're interested in how long we can keep animals alive, with metastatic advanced stage 4 cancers. We have a different outcome, different perspective on looking at this whole thing.

But yeah, we have achieved levels of success that are beyond anything we would have ever expected. Without toxicity! And that's diet drug cocktails, that will work just great.

We published a big paper on this, called The Press Pulse Therapeutic Strategy, with some of my clinician colleagues. It outlines the framework for how we would treat human cancers with the press pulse therapeutic strategy.

The diet is the press - and then we use strategic drugs, with the diet, to pulse them. Not chronically use them, but pulse the drugs. And that slowly degrades the tumor, while enhancing the health and vitality of the normal cells.

Many cancer patients who come into the clinic, they not only have cancer, they often have diabetes, they often have some other comorbidities associated with the fact that they have cancer.

In our metabolic press pulse strategies, we not only manage the cancer, reducing it significantly. But we also get rid of the diabetes, we get rid of the hypertension, we get rid of the other comorbidities that these patients also have had.

Clearly: Linking all of these chronic diseases to a common underlying provocative situation - which is nutritional imbalance. Diets and treatments that provoke the growth of these tumors, and persist on these kinds of conditions.

So clearly, once you understand the biology of the problem, the solutions become much, much more clear and logical.

Dr. Chaffee:

Yeah. I was going to say, too, about the radiation: Obviously, we do use this in the pediatric populations. It can be absolutely devastating to those kids.

I think that if I were in a position... even not knowing the things that we're talking about now. I don't think I would ever let my child get radiation for a tumor.

Prof. Seyfried:

You might not have a choice.

Dr. Chaffee:

What?

Prof. Seyfried:

You might not have a choice! Because if that child is lower than 16 years of age or 18, the system determines what you should do to that child.

Dr. Chaffee:

Oh, really?

Prof. Seyfried:

The system determines. The parents are taken out of the equation. Unless... Remember, the woman that went to mexico to save the life of her child?

The system controls what you do to that child. So even if you said the standard of care involves radiation and chemo for that child, it's very hard to break the system. They'll have you arrested as 'parental neglect'.

That's what I'm talking about: The system is very powerful.

Dr. Chaffee:
That's definitely too much! I've seen kids who have grown up after getting radiation like this, it completely stuns their mental development. So where wherever were, it probably damaged them from that point...

Say, they're three, they damaged them from three - and then they never develop past that.

So you have this person in this 30-year old body, with the mind of a 5-year-old. Or less. And it's absolutely tragic to see that.

Prof. Seyfried:
More tragic is: It doesn't have to happen!

Dr. Chaffee:
Yeah, exactly.

Prof. Seyfried:
That doesn't have to happen, that's the tragedy. That child could have been rescued. I'm not saying the child could have been cured, but if the child lives to be the same age, they would be cognitively intact. Not cognitively challenged.

Dr. Chaffee:
Yeah, and we talk about quality of life and we do give people the choice:

Is this something that you want to do? Given the fact that this is going to be a pretty rough road. Do you want to just live out your last months at a better standard of living? Or go for the gold?

I think that especially when you're talking about about a child who could potentially have such devastating damage to their brain and their development, for me, I would never want that personally - and I don't think I would ever want that for my child either.

Prof. Seyfried:
No, no one does. But this is the way it is. And you often see the child...

They're given such high dose steroids, they get the big moon face. The steroids are driving blood sugars to extremely high levels. Then once you see that phenotype, the big moon face -

whether it's in a child or an adult with a glioblastoma – you know they're finished.

You know that the therapy itself is killing those people. That's the tragedy.

What I just said to you, that statement that I just made, is not known to the majority of practitioners in the field: They are under the impression that this is helping their patient! This is the gap in knowledge that needs to be closed.

We cannot continue to do this toxic therapy on these poor people. Whether it's a child or an adult. It speaks to the lack of knowledge on the part of the field treating a disease. Okay?

It has to change. It has to change, otherwise we have to continue to see these tragedies one after another. Not only in America, throughout the world. You're in Australia, they're doing the same thing down there as we do here. In England, Germany, Japan. They're all doing the same thing.

It's a worldwide tragedy! And it will only change once everybody comes to realize that cancer is a mitochondrial metabolic disease. We could make a dent in this disease so quick, if people knew what I just said.

The problem is: They don't want to know about it, they don't want to hear about it, they don't want to talk about it. For various reasons.

Dr. Chaffee:
On that note: You mentioned there are some clinics and centers that are using this as a model. Where are these guys at and how are they getting away with it?

Prof. Seyfried:
Well, I think there's small clinics that have patients... they have to be offered an alternative. Right now, if you go to the main hospitals like Dana-Farber, MD Anderson, Sloan Kettering, wherever else they have these major cancer centers, they're not offering metabolic therapy.

Doctors should offer metabolic therapy, see with the patients. The problem is: If you're going to be Dana-Farber or MD Anderson and you want to do metabolic therapy - there's no one there really that knows what to do!

You have to have a staff of professionals that know what to do, and how to do it! Okay? Without that knowledge base, it's not going to work.

Even worse: The young people going through medical schools in the oncology area, they're not trained to do metabolic therapy. So where is the training coming from?

We have written a protocol to treat cancer patients, based on metabolic therapy. With Miriam Kalamian, a world-renowned expert on keto for cancer and diet for this. She's helped a lot of cancer patients.

We wrote a treatment protocol. Can it be used? It will not be used in the major hospitals, of course. Because you're doing it as an alternative to radiation, chemo, immunotherapies and these other kinds of things.

But it can be done in smaller clinics. In smaller clinics that are not so yoked by the system, to do what they have to do.

The goal is to keep people alive - and have the people themselves tell everyone this is what I did. Guy Tenenbaum, he's on the web, overcame his stage 4 prostate cancer using metabolic approaches!

So you're getting more and more vocal advocates that are telling others that, "Listen, do metabolic therapy!" Now, is it easy? I don't want to let people think that doing metabolic therapy is a cakewalk.

Because a lot of the success rides on your shoulders: How compliant are you to not eat carbohydrates - which can be very hard for a lot of people.

Dr. Chaffee:
Yeah. That's one of the things I see in clinic, here in neurosurgery:

We get these people with the GBMs, this devastating diagnosis.

I think every single patient that I've ever done a consultation with... and we do this once a week, we have everyone come in with all the new diagnoses. And I don't think there's a single person that hasn't asked me "Okay, what can I do? How can I do this?" They don't want to feel helpless, but it is just out of their control.

And I remember getting really upset at another physician. They asked him, sort of "Well, should I stop eating sugar? Should I stop drinking alcohol? Or what should I do?" - and the doctor's like "You know what? You probably don't have that long anyway, so just do whatever you want."

I was so furious at that!

Prof. Seyfried:

Yeah.

Dr. Chaffee:

The person looked so defeated, he was like "Yeah, I guess it just doesn't matter." I was like "Of course it matters! It absolutely matters! You have control, you have a say in this. You have a dog in this fight, you are able to affect your own course of your life!"

And just seeing their eyes, literally hope just rising in their eyes... and I try to mitigate that because this isn't good any way you cut it.

But I tell them: I tell them about your work, I point them in the direction of your material and studies, and I just say:

"Hey look, I'm not telling you that this is going to cure anything, it's not going to stop anything. But there's a lot of evidence that says that if you do this, this will help. Here, just go to the source. See what you think.

Prof. Seyfried:

You're 100% correct about that and I can't emphasize that more than what you just said. Because I see people... once they understand about the glucose ketone index, measuring their own blood every day - not every day, but every other day or whatever, using a little meter.

And they're collecting the numbers and they know what direction those numbers have to go, for that therapy to be effective – with that, they get really motivated!

They now know that they are able to do something. They are in control of their own destiny. And they work very hard and they become extremely motivated!

This is what Pablo did: When he knew what numbers he had to achieve in order to put pressure on the growth of that tumor, he knew he was in control.

You give the patient now power, they have the power and they get motivated to know what they need to do. You're absolutely right: Nobody should ever be told there's nothing more we can do.

Especially at the beginning of their disease. Then they have to know that it's a long haul. It's not like I'm really good at this for a month.

No, no. You're gonna have to bite the bullet on this and power it through, until you have achieved control of that growth. The growth does not control you, control the growth of the cancer.

Dr. Chaffee:

Yeah!

Prof. Seyfried:

The patient can do that with the proper motivation, with the proper training. So I can't emphasize more what you just said. You've got to let these patients know that they're part of the fight and they can control this.

You'd be surprised how much longer these people live, in a higher quality of life. And when they... I don't want to say they all pass. But I've had people tell me, or their loved ones, told me that "This guy fought the fight. He felt so good about himself - and even though he may not have made it all the way, he lived 2, 3 times longer than he was supposed to live - at a much higher quality of life! And never had to suffer and die in these painful situations."

Then there's many people who are still fighting the fight and should have died a long time ago, and they're still on!

If I had the drugs that work with the diet, we would be able to settle this in a much more defined period of time. So yeah, there's a lot of hope for the future.

I would say the future of cancer is bright, not bleak! You know, it's a whole new strategy and I think that the future of cancer is: We can keep this disease managed and people are going to emerge in a healthier state and feel much better about themselves.

That's my view. I base it on my understanding of the biology of the disease, and 30 years of research in the field, looking at this problem. And publishing all these papers. This is the way I see it.

I think the future is far brighter than it should be, than people make it out to be.

Dr. Chaffee:

Yeah, good! I agree with you! Just trying to get this out there and let people know that they actually have a say in this. hen they can actually affect the course of this disease. They're not just out of control and just at the whims of the chemo and radiation - but they actually have something to say in this as well.

When did you get this focus in your line of research? I know that when you were at Yale, you were doing research on seizures and preventing seizures with ketosis.

Which is something that I've looked into. And it's like, we've been using this for nearly 90 years to treat refractory seizures. But yet, it's something that almost no neurologist that I know of uses.

I've seen a lot of people with epilepsy, have spoken to them. I always ask them have they ever spoken to you about your diet? Not a single one has said yes.

Which just blows my mind! Because it's such a simple thing. It may not be easy to implement, but it is straightforward, and it has a lot of evidence behind it.

Prof. Seyfried:
Well, don't forget: At that time, Yale was one of the leaders in the field of epilepsy research. Gilbert Glaser was the chair of the department. Had written many, many distinguished books and papers on epilepsy.

And they told me... because I was working on ganglioside biochemistry at the time, looking at different disorders of lipid metabolism. But they said: "If you want to stay at Yale, you better work on something to do with epilepsy."

So we were mapping genes for epileptic seizures. Everybody was excited mapping genes. Because the idea was if you map the gene, you could figure out the product and you can make a treatment for that product.

Then I realized that we always tried to do the same kind of chemicals and things all the time - why don't we try keto? I didn't do ketogenic diet until I came to Boston.

I tried to get a grant at Yale, but they said nobody's interested in ketogenic diets for epilepsy, we have all these drugs. But then Jim Abrams of the movie industry, produced the film First do no harm with Meryl Streep - his son charlie had epilepsy. He started the Charlie Foundation.

He brought together a lot of people in the epilepsy field to look at: Why are we not using ketogenic diets to manage epilepsy, when it was known since by 1921 by Wilder at Mayo Clinic? Why are we not doing this?

So one of my students went out to the meeting, we were still doing looking at epilepsy. She came back and said "Hey listen!
130

We should put our mice on ketogenic diets!" And sure enough... we had mapped all these genes, but the thing was the diet blocked the seizures. It was really quite an interesting thing.

Then calorie restriction was even more powerful, along with ketogenic diets. And then we were working on the gangliosides for brain cancer, we were doing a lot of work on brain cancer.

Then we said "Why don't we see if the diet works on brain cancer?" After the results, I said "Oh my god, this is unbelievable! What's going on here?!" Then we discovered Otto Warburg had said this many, many years ago.

We know that the tumors can't burn ketones for energy because their mitochondria are defective, they need glucose. So when the glucose is low and the ketones are elevated, the tumors shrink. Makes perfect sense, Otto Warburg was right!

That then send us off into a better understanding of how we manage cancer metabolically, coming from our understanding of how ketogenic diets work on epileptic seizures.

Actually, we still don't know the mechanism by which ketogenic diets block epilepsy, because it's a very complicated brain wiring scenario that has to be looked into. But it became crystal clear as how this diet could stop cancer growth, or restrict cancer growth.

The fact is that we have tens of thousands of little kids around the world, using ketogenic diets every day to manage their seizures. Yet, when you talk about it in cancer, they go "Oh, it could hurt the kid, it could hurt the patient! The toxic effects of ketogenic diets,"

What? Are you kidding me? We have thousands of little kids doing ketogenic diets for epilepsy, and nobody's talking about that - but when you take a little kid with cancer oh no, terribly toxic, it's nutritionally impalanced...

What? Are you nuts? Compared to radiation and chemo? You're telling me that a ketogenic diet is more harmful than radiation and chemo? I mean, give me a break

Dr. Chaffee:
Exactly!

Prof. Seyfried:
This is the absurdity of dealing with the field. We came to this state where we are through a long, circuitous path. Not knowing where any of this would have ever ever taken us. But we were

aware enough of the underlying mechanisms of action to know what we were doing, why we were doing it, and how it works.

Now the big challenge is getting the word out to people and seeing more and more success stories of using this. Now in Los Angeles, a collegue of mine has a big trial with ketogenic diet for glioblastoma.

And he's getting spectacular results, more than he would have ever imagined. But that's still with upfront standard of care! He and I know... I said "If you took away that radiation and chemo, your results would probably be even more spectacular."

So it just takes time for the system to come to adjust and realize what's happening here. There is a very clear mechanism of action. So it just takes time, that's all.

But I feel that this current time is being wasted, and we're sacrificing all these poor kids and adults to cancer, that's the tragedy. That this doesn't have to happen and yet, it's happening.

Dr. Chaffee:

So these damaged mitochondria: Obviously, this is precipitating this issue. Can that ever reverse? Or is there always be a point of no return... but does that ever come back? Meaning the status of healthy mitochondria.

Prof. Seyfried:

Well, that was one of the big things that I did when I bundled together all the nuclear mitochondrial transfer experiments that were done in animal systems over decades.

All independent of each other, done by some of the best developmental biologists in the field, and I spoke to some of these individuals.

If you take the nucleus of the tumor cell that has all the mutations that are supposedly drivers, and you drop that nucleus into a new cytoplasm, you get growth regulation! Not growth dysregulation.

And sometimes you can form a whole frog or a mouse from the nucleus of a tumor cell. So you replaced essentially the bad mitochondria. In other words you put that nucleus into a cytoplasm with fresh mitochondria - and those new mitochondria are able to re-regulate the growth and development.

Despite the continued presence of the so-called driver gene mutations that we're supposed to... I mean, this is the hardest evidence against this gene theory.

If you do the reverse, if you take the normal nucleus and drop it into a cytoplasm that has cancerous mitochondria, the cell will either die or form dysregulated cancer cells. This is clear evidence.

Getting back to your question: Can we revert cancer by putting new mitochondria in there. It's called mitochondrial therapy, actually. I think that's gonna come in the future.

I think it's so new that eventually we will be able to maybe replace them. But I don't want to, at this point, say "Let's see if we can restore the growth regulation of a cancer cell by putting in new mitochondria."

I think it's better at this point to kill them off, get rid of them! Put them in a growth lock hold, rather than trying to re-educate them. I think mitochondrial therapy for the future is going to be really exciting and interesting.

I don't think we're there yet. So let's work with what we can do, and make a real big difference. Then we'll move forward with these newer kinds of therapies for the future.

But right now, let's just put a lock hold on these cancer cells and keep people alive in a healthier state. If that means eating tomahawk ribeyes, I think you'll find a number of people that would buy on to that.

Dr. Chaffee:
Yeah. That experiment that you spoke of, taking the nucleus and then putting it into a new cytoplasm and the mitochondria - showing that you have all these genetic changes and it doesn't behave as cancer. And you take the mitochondria and put them in - and it does behave as cancer! That's qed, as far as I'm concerned.

Prof. Seyfried:
Yeah, but it's still... The response by the oncology field is: They don't want to talk about it, they don't want to look at it and they don't want to hear about it!

That's because it's so devastating to an entire industry. That, once that becomes more widely recognized...

Dr. Chaffee:
Yeah.

Prof. Seyfried:

...and it's been repeated over and over, in all different different kinds of models. So what's the holdup? What is the holdup here?

Somebody has to scratch their head and say "What? Why do we continue to persist with therapies, that put patients at risk for all kinds of health diseases, when we have a solution, a better approach, to management than we currently have?"

What is the holdup here? [Laughter]

Dr. Chaffee:

So if someone were to have cancer now, what would be the best way to manage it? Obviously, going ketogenic or even carnivore. What ratio are they looking for to get?

Like, what is so the best way for people to manage this at home, if they don't have access to one of these clinics that are popping up?

Prof. Seyfried:

Well, as I said in the letters that I sent to people, I'm not a physician. I can't tell you what to do and what not to do.

All I can do is provide you with information, knowledge, from published papers and observations. And I'll let the physicians in the clinics treat the patients.

We know what we need to do, see the press pulse paper. Now, a lot of people cannot do water-only fasting because it's too much of a shock. The brain is addicted to glucose. And it's it's just as difficult to get off glucose than it is to get off heroin, alcohol and nicotine, these kinds of things.

But the body can adjust to the change. So, you will have withdrawal symptoms. What we realized is that if the patient were to gradually transition to a zero carbohydrate diet, for several weeks - even that can be difficult for some patients...

But it's not as much of a jump to doing a water-only fast. I tried it, man! Going cold turkey on carbs is really, really tough! I mean, you can smell stuff cooking like blocks away.

Dr. Chaffee:

Haha!

Prof. Seyfried:

It's unbelievable! It's too hard. What we've learned is that patients can transition to water-only fasting after a couple of weeks on zero carb diets. With meat, no carbs at all. Some vegetables, we're not as opposed to veggies as you might be.

But if we can get organically grown vegetables... grow them in your backyard, using manure and these kinds of things.

I tell you, then the transition to water-only fasting for a few days is way easier. Bring those blood sugars down, bring the ketones up. Get into the new diet state, then you hit him with the drugs. A drug like DON and some of the other drugs.

There are all these parasite medications. Man, they're really damn powerful!

Yeah, you hit them with Mebendazole, Fenbendazole, they target some of the metabolic pathways that the cancer cells need.

Dr. Chaffee:

Okay!

Prof. Seyfried:

All this stuff is cheap. Now here's the interesting thing...

And Bendazole was really cheap, it's a parasite medication. For some sort of worms. You can get the pills over in India for 50 cents a tablet.

But now, when we realized in the United States these medications work with cancer treatment, it's 300 dollars a tablet!

Dr. Chaffee:

Aww! Come on!

Prof. Seyfried:

Yeah, you tell me what's the drive in this industry. It's not helping, it's revenue generation.

You know the guy Martin Shkreli, the most hated man in America? Who made the EpiPens like 800 dollars?

Dr. Chaffee:

Right!

Prof. Seyfried:

Remember that guy? He took advantage of the system because he could. Everybody hated the guy. But the pharmaceutical industry does the same thing, they just don't broadcast it. It's now called shkreli, you shkreli the price of all these things you can make a buck on.

Dr. Chaffee:

Haha!

Prof. Seyfried:

It's terrible, right? It's really despicable behavior.

Dr. Chaffee:

It is!

Prof. Seyfried:

Yeah, but that's the business of America.

These are the drugs. You can get drugs on the cheap, as long as know how to use them. You put them together with diet drug combinations, and you can get a really good powerful management of cancer.

But you have to have knowledgeable people. They have to know doses, timing and scheduling. This is all quite doable, the framework is already here, we published the framework. So, if people are willing to know how to do this, they're willing to take it, they should follow that framework.

Cancer patients, sure, they can do a lot of it themselves - as long as they're educated and told what to do and how to do it.

Then you have non-invasive imaging technology that can monitor their cancer, to see whether or not it's growing. Whether or not it's stabilized - or whether or not it's still there or not.

We don't need to be taking punch biopsies and doing all this crazy stuff. What are you doing biopsies for?

Everybody's like "Oh, I gotta have a biopsy of my cancer." Why? "I don't know if it's malignant." Well, if it's malignant, you should never take a punch biopsy, you could spread it all over the damn body!

And if it's a benign, what the are hell you sticking a benign tumor for? So they want to get a gene profile of the cells that come out of your tumor - to tell you what kind of a new drug, a new toxic drug, that will target that mutation you should take.

But: The damn cells are using glucose and glutamine! Why don't you target that before you stick the tumor?!

I mean, everything we're doing is like back ass forward. You got to know what to do, how to do it. Educate people, educate the practitioners - and things will begin to change. They have to change, we can't continue to do what we're doing.

Dr. Chaffee:

I completely agree. Professor Seyfried, thank you so much for coming on. I really appreciate it, it's been an absolute pleasure to speak with you.

I've been referencing your work and pointing people towards you for a number of years now. I really appreciate this opportunity to speak with you, so thank you very much!

Prof. Seyfried:

Well, thank you. I hope some of this information can help people.

And our support that we have comes from philanthropy and private foundations.

Obviously, there are people who recognize what we are doing, what we are saying and the strategies.

There are good people! Who say you're doing the right thing let me support what you're doing. Because it's very hard to get the federal government granting system funds, through the National Cancer Institute - when everybody thinks cancer is a genetic disease. And you're coming along, telling them "It's not!"

You don't go very far in getting funds for doing that kind of stuff. But yeah, we'll keep pushing. We have the best pre-clinical model systems, the best trained staff a knowledgeable staff - and we're not going anywhere.

Dr. Chaffee:
Good!

Prof. Seyfried:
We're pushing forward on this until the job is done. So thanks for reading, I hope this helps your audience.

Dr. Chaffee:
Well, I hope it does too. And there are certainly people that are suffering from cancer or they will become afflicted by it. I think anyone who reads this and knows someone with cancer, I really encourage them to borrrow them this book - so that they can really understand what's going on.

Actually, so that they can really understand, that they have a lot more to say in their own prognosis and recovery than they might think they do!

Professor Seyfried, what's the best place for people to find you and find your work? You mentioned your email that you send out to people. Is there a link to a website or something?

Prof. Seyfried:
Yes, there's a link to the Foundation For Cancer Metabolic Therapies, we obtain money from private foundations.
People can also support us through Boston College, they can send funds directly to my research program.

Dr. Chaffee:
Okay!

Prof. Seyfried:

These kinds of things. And believe it or not, more and more people are coming out to support this. Because it's going to have a greater impact in supporting almost anything else in the cancer field, there's no question about that.

So the faster we get our papers published, the more evidence we continue to accumulate... case reports, human case reports: We do that!

So I help the physicians to write up the case reports on the patients that have survived longer than than would be expected. It takes a lot of my time, of course, but I'm willing to do this.

And our peer-reviewed scientific publications continue to push this field forward.

This requires funding to do because we have to pay lots of things. There's animal costs, staff costs, consumables. Things that we use, equipment costs, things to maintain...

Bottom line is: Yeah, I send a letter out that has information, helps cancer patients make decisions, try to get them with the right contacts. People who understand what's going on, and then they take it from there.

This has been the plan so far. It seems to be gaining more and more momentum, as more and more word gets out about this whole cancer thing. And things begin to change.

Dr. Chaffee:
Fantastic! I encourage people to go, visit and to donate. I think that this sort of work is really important.

Prof. Seyfried:
The letters that I send out... it's only asking for a donation if you feel that that information helps you. If something helps you, you might consider a donation. I am not asking anybody... only if the information that I send is of value. I don't charge anything for this.

The bottom line is to see the results, more than anything else. I think that's the most important thing at this stage.

Dr. Chaffee:
I completely agree. There's a lot of things that I don't get paid for as well. I stay late, talk to people. And talk to people outside of the hospital, to try and get them better.

Because that's why we're here! You know, I think a lot of people, a lot of doctors and researchers are still in that mindset

- but unfortunately, some have forgotten that. Or forgotten that it's even possible to do that anymore.

Prof. Seyfried:
Yeah. Anyway, I'll let you go. Thank you very much and thank you for the interview.

Dr. Chaffee:
Thank you, I really appreciate it.

Chapter 5: Controversial Interview, The Drive #30; With Dr. Peter Attia

Hello everyone! Welcome to this week's episode of the Peter Attia Drive. My guest this week is Professor Tom Seyfried, who many of you will know - but I suspect an equal number of you will not know.

Tom has come to us through many channels, meaning the requests to speak with Tom have come on many levels. There's been a lot of requests through social media, through the site and of course based on our discussions with Dom D'Agostino. Dom has been friend of mine for quite a while.

This is my first time meeting Tom, but I feel like I know him because I've read so much of his work.

Tom's background is that he's got a PhD in genetics and biochemistry from the University of Illinois, got that in the mid 70s. He did his postdoc in the Department of Neurology at Yale.

It was there, that he first became interested in ketones because of their application in the amelioration of recalcitrant seizures. As we get into in the episode, that led to his interest in cancer, which is now his focus.

Tom has published over 150 peer-reviewed publications. He's the author of numerous books, textbooks etc., including kind of a treatise on this. His magnum opus is effectively a book called

Cancer as a Metabolic Disease.

I got my copy of this a few years ago and in many ways, that's why felt quite familiar in speaking with him.

He's currently a professor at Boston College, and his research today focuses on the mechanisms by which metabolic therapies can manage chronic diseases such as epilepsy, neurodegenerative lipid storage diseases... and above all: Cancer.

In this episode, we talk about Tom's background, his work in epilepsy and how that led him to the interest in caloric restriction and ketosis.

We revisit the man, the legend, Otto Warburg and talk about the Warburg Effect and Warburg's point of view on these things...

...and I do push him a little bit on this. Because I want to point out that it's not entirely clear amongst people what the Warburg Effect really implies and how ubiquitous it is.

I have to be honest with you: I don't necessarily share Tom's views on a number of these things. So I wanted to do my best to represent as many other views as possible. But at the same time, I hope the discussion is helpful.

We get into a bunch of the semantics. I knew this was a very technical topic and I know that not everybody has the luxury of listening to this, while they're reviewing the show notes. We do go over the difference between respiration or oxidative phosphorylation and fermentation.

We also get into this idea of substrate level phosphorylation - a very important concept - and the fermentation of glucose.

We also talk a lot about glutamine. This is something that I haven't spent a lot of time talking about in the past. I think I do touch on it a little bit with Dom D'Agostino, but we get into it in much greater fashion jere.

Of course we get into the ultimately fundamental question.
Which is:

- *Is cancer primarily a metabolic disease? Meaning a disease whose origin arrives in the mitochondria or in the metabolic machinery of the cell*
- *Or is it primarily a genetic disease where sometimes you will and sometimes you won't sustain mitochondrial damage?*

Now, you'll see this in the interview, it's not entirely clear to me that I buy the argument, that cancer is entirely a metabolic disease. Though as some of you will know, I am very bullish on the use of metabolic therapies in cancer. But I'm also very bullish on the use of immunotherapy in cancer. And, when appropriate, chemotherapy in cancer.

My view is that cancer is about as hard a disease as there is ever going to be to target, therefore we ought to turn our attention to as many legs of the stool as possible and not just one.

The discussion gets a little bit heated at one point, when I take issue with something Tom said about suggesting that biopsies could exacerbate cancer. I really don't want anybody to come out of this, believing that having a biopsy is going to increase their risk of metastatic cancer.

I think that anyone's entitled to a hypothesis. But, to my knowledge, there is absolutely no evidence to support that claim.

We talk a lot about a particular type of cancer called glioblastoma multiforme, GBM. Also known as a grade 4 astrocytoma. This is a cancer that, if you haven't heard of it, you've certainly heard of its effect.

John McCain, who recently passed away, suffered from this. I lost a friend to this when I was younger... and I think that if you know somebody who has died of brain cancer, there's a pretty good chance this is the cancer they had.

This is one of those cancers that gives cancer a bad name. In all fairness, I don't think there's ever been a true documented survivor of this cancer. It also may provide one of the more interesting model systems to study metabolic therapies for cancer.

I guess the most important thing we close with is: I sort of pushed Tom a little bit on what experiment he would want to see or do to advance the thinking in this field.

In many ways, Tom's a little bit of a guy that's on the sidelines of mainstream cancer.

These views, these metabolic views unfortunately don't get the attention they deserve. And other people that I'm going to be talking with in the future, such as Sid Mukherjee and Lew Cantley are going to be some of the people who are now starting to see, through their own research, some of the potential applications for these things.

So I think that in many ways, the problems that Tom has been working on for the last 30 or 40 years, are very slowly beginning to gain acceptance in the more mainstream circles of oncology.

With that said, please give it up for my guest today, Dr. Tom Seyfried:

Dr. Peter Attia:
Hey Tom, how are you?
Prof. Thomas Seyfried:
Fine! Thank you very much.
Dr. Attia:
Well, thank you so much for making time. I know you've got a long lineup of students outside your office, who are angry at me for sitting here, taking up time - when you could be answering their questions.
Prof. Seyfried:
They'll recover.
Dr. Attia:
Haha! A lot of people have been reaching out to me on social media, saying you've got to have Tom on, you've got to have Tom on the podcast. The one with Don was excellent but there's so much more we want to understand about cancer.

And certainly, cancer is something near and dear to my heart. I did my fellowship in oncology. But at the same time, I think I understand cancer far less than I understand things that I didn't formally got trained in. Like I think I have a better understanding for example of heart disease than I do of cancer.

So I'm really excited to explore a lot of topics today... and acknowledge that we probably won't even scratch the surface of all that you know and think about.

But all that said: How did you get interested in this?

Prof. Seyfried:

Well, we started it when I was at Yale University, the Department of Neurology. Where we had been working on epilepsy, lipid storage diseases and gangliosides, basically. Complex lipid molecules.

And one of the individuals that I was working with at that time, Robert Hugh - he was my mentor at the time. He had done some research on ganglioside changes in tumors, and we had been looking at that. There were some interesting molecules in those tumor cells.

I also knew Dennis Spencer, who was the chief of neurosurgery at the time at Yale. He said „Why don't you come up to the operating room with me and I'll get you a nice piece of glioblastoma from a patient?“ You know, I'm a basic scientist, I'm not a clinician, I don't know what's going on. So I said „Sure!“

In the operating room, that was kind of an experience that I'll never forget. Having someone take a tumor out of someone's head.

And they were asking me all kinds of questions, like „Do you think we should put pellets of radiation in the cavity?“ all this kind of stuff. I didn't know, I said „I'm here to look at the ganglioside pattern in the tumor, I don't treat the cancer or anything like this.“

But in any event, we had then started making our own brain tumors in the mouse, based on the work of Harry Zimmerman. Who started the first school of neuropathology in the United States at Yale University, back in the 1930s. He was still alive at the time, he lived to be 98 years old.

So I was interested in doing comparative studies of glycolipids in human- and mouse brain tumors, to see whether or not we can come to some common changes. That's how we got started, pretty much looking at comparative biochemical profiles between human tumors and mouse tumors.

There were some similarities, but there were many differences as well. But we didn't get into the kind of therapeutic evaluation of these tumors.

We also had a huge program in epilepsy, mapping genes for epilepsy. We did a lot of things at Yale, working on the glycolipids of the tumors, glycolipids of developing brain. Lipid storage diseases and epilepsy.

And... I wrote a grant, internally at Yale - which was rejected.

Asking about ketogenic diets.

Dr. Attia:

What year was this?

Prof. Seyfried:

This was back in the late 70s, early 80s maybe. 1980. And they said „Oh, nobody's interested in ketogenic diets. It's kind of passé."

Dr. Attia:

This was before the work at Hopkins?

Prof. Seyfried:

Yeah, Hopkins... John Freeman was a friend of mine, too. Who was the Godfather of ketogenic diets. He was the one that saved Jim Abram's son Charlie.

Jim was a movie director. And his friend Meryl Streep made the movie First, do no harm - which was in part based on Jim's experience with his son. But I wasn't connected at that time to Abrams or any of that stuff, that was even before the Charlie Foundation.

I just had this inkling that maybe ketogenic diet would be interesting to test against some of the epilepsy models that I was working with.

Dr. Attia:

Does that mean you suspected that epilepsy had something to do with glucose metabolism?

Prof. Seyfried:

No, not at all. I just thought it was an interesting approach, a non-drug approach for seizures.

Anyway, the grant was summarily rejected. I said „Well, nobody's interested in this." So I left Yale and I came up to Boston College here, start a program.

And then we were here. From then, it was 10 years, 15 years later, we developed some of the best animal models for epilepsy. We were looking at the brains, at the biochemistry of epileptic seizures and the genes that caused epilepsy.

Then one of my PhD students, Marianna Tran said „Oh, they're having a big meeting out in Washington on ketogenic diets for epilepsy. Maybe our model would be appropriate for this!" I said „Nah..."

After my experience at Yale, I said nobody's interested in this crap anyway, haha.

Dr. Attia:
You were still traumatized by the grant thing.

Prof. Seyfried:
Right! Anyway, I had a few extra bucks in the grant, so I said „Okay, go on out." In fact, she wrote a little blurb and they funded her to go out there.

She comes back and starts telling me „Wow, you can't believe what I saw out there! All these guys are interested in ketogenic diets! This guy, Jim Abrams, he told us about this foundation called the Charly Foundation - and it was to study epilepsy and ketogenic diets!"

I said „All right, what the hell..." So we started to put that on the mice! It was funny, because we didn't know what we were doing. But then at the same time... two things came together at the same time:

We were studying gangliosides for lipid storage diseases. There was a drug company over in England that gave us this new drug that was supposed to stop gangliosides synthesis, and therefore reduced the storage in the brain.

At that time at Boston College, they didn't charge me for animals - which they do now. Which is a tragedy! Because you can really do a lot of work... the damn mice cost so much money.

And there were so fewer restrictions. I mean, we followed all of the animal care protocols. Back then, we had access to a large number, so we could do experiments that you couldn't do anywhere else.

So when we got the drug from the company, we were feeding the drug to the mice, and we looked at the gangliosides, „Yeah, it's really down!" But: So was the body weight!

Then, when we put the control group in, we found out that, yes, the tumors shrunk and the gangliosides were reduced from this drug - but the body weight was also reduced.

Dr. Attia:
Were both animals being fed ad lib?

Prof. Seyfried:
Yes, ad libitum. One had the drug, one didn't.
Dr. Attia:
Okay. So the drug somehow either reduced caloric intake or increased expenditure.
Prof. Seyfried:
We don't know, but the body weights were reduced by about 15 to 20%. And the tumors were significantly reduced, by about 50, 60%!

So I told the company... it was just a pilot study. I told the company „Your drug seems to really shrink brain tumors." They go „What?! This is a much bigger market!" - than, say, Tay–Sachs disease.

That's when they gave me $200,000 to investigate the mechanism by which their drug was stopping brain cancer. Because I showed them the data, and they were all excited.

So we then began to investigate this, with Dr. Mukarjee. I hired her specifically to start looking at this. Then, when we realized that what's working...

She said „A lot of times, these drugs work through calorie restriction". So I said „Why don't we put a control group?"

We all decided: Let's put a control group for body weights. One was the guys with the drug and losing weight - with the other guys, we would just take the food away from them. So the body weights would be absolutely identical.
Dr. Attia:
So they were pair fed?
Prof. Seyfried:
No, it wasn't pair fed. One group was eating ad libitum and they were losing body weight. And the other group, we had to restrict the calories to match the body weight
Dr. Attia:
So they were pair weighted?
Prof. Seyfried:
Pair weighted, yes. Then we evaluated this - and the tumors were exactly the same size! So it had nothing to do with the drug, even though the drug was working on the targeted molecule, it wasn't the targeted molecule that was responsible for this.

That's when we also decided... with the epilepsy, overlapping: Does the ketogenic diet work through calorie restriction?
146

Because many of these children that get ketogenic diets, they have very restricted calories.

You can't let kids eat massive amounts of fat. Because invariably... John Freeman told me, the diet doesn't work if they just let them eat all the fat they want. Some kids just love to eat all this fat, and then the seizures don't go away.

Dr. Attia:
In other words: The thinking at the time was that there is some amount of caloric restriction that is necessary, within the context of the ketosis, to also affect the epileptic seizures.

Prof. Seyfried:
Yes, absolutely. But you have to be very careful because many of these children are on the growth spurt - so you have to be careful on how much restriction you give.

The other thing of course is it's self restricted: There's several physiological systems in our body that, when you eat a lot of fat, you just don't need a lot of calories. It's a turn-off. It works through the vagus nerve.

The hormone cholecystokinin is kind of an appetite suppressor. It affects the vagus nerve, which then stops the appetite. You don't eat as much.

I have so many stories, so I was sitting on a bus one day...

Dr. Attia:
You're on the right podcast, we don't have any time restrictions here!

Prof. Seyfried:
Yeah, great! Listen: So they made this thing called the vagal nerve stimulator. It was made by a company, I can't remember the name of it. They made a fortune!

They would implant the stimulator into the person who has epilepsy and it would send out things to stimulate the vagus nerve.

And I was sitting on the bus with this guy from Norway, and I say

„Are you putting this into the patient?"

„Yeah, we sort of put this into the patient."

„How does it work?"

„Yeah, it seems to work really good."

I said „How much is it?" He says „Well, the operation is like 4,000 dollars. But the device itself, it's 15,000 dollars." They were

147

putting them in all these epileptic patients. I asked „how does it work?!" He said „I don't know, but it works!"

I didn't know, I'm just sitting on the bus, I don't know. We're going to MGM studios down in Florida. They closed the whole place down in the middle of the week in December, so that they could attract all the epileptologists to use their device to put into these patients. It's one of these kind of things...

Anyway, when we were working on ketogenic diets and calorie restriction: We realized that humans have this internal system to stop ingesting calories. And if you don't stop the calories, invariably, you don't get the management of the seizures.

So we, in our parallel studies in epilepsy with mice and cancer and all this other stuff, we started to learn what's working in the patients. How do we translate what's working in the patients into the mice? The mice can be another source of information that we can feed back.

We published this big paper on calorie restriction and that the ketogenic diet was working largely through calorie restriction - and maintaining low blood sugar levels was the key to maintaining control of seizures.

Dr. Attia:
I don't know if you did this experiment, but if you took animals on an equally low caloric diet that was not ketogenic... So let's just say a very high carbohydrate, low fat diet, where presumably glucose levels would be higher, even though they would still be calorically restricted - would you get the same anti-seizure benefit?

Prof. Seyfried:
The same results. Exactly. Because what was happening is that when the body is restricted of calories, you then make ketones. So the level of ketosis was also seen in the calorie restricted mice. It was like a human doing water only fasting.

Dr. Attia:
So how calorically restricted did they need to be, if they were not on a ketogenic diet?

Prof. Seyfried:
A 35 to 40 percent restriction. Then we did some studies, another group:

We found out that 35 to 40% restriction of calories in the mouse equates to a water only therapeutic fasting in humans.

148

That's because the their metabolism is 7 or 8 times higher than that of a man. So humans can achieve much higher ketosis than a mouse can.

A one day water-only fast in a mouse is like a 7-day water only fast in a human, and the blood sugars go down, the ketones go up.

Dr. Attia:
IRBs [Institutional review boards] don't allow you to fast mice that long anymore, do they?

Prof. Seyfried:
Oh yeah! As long as they're healthy. Calorie restriction is generally a healthy thing. You don't want to over restrict because then you're put into nutritional imbalance, and you don't want to go to a level of what we call starvation. Calorie restriction is healthy, up to the point where you start breaking down muscle.

If you start breaking down muscle, then you enter into a new physiological state called starvation and that's very pathological. You don't ever want to go to that digression. Some people get so carried away with water only fasting, they can enter into starvation mode.

I know this for a fact because I used to spend a lot of time with George Cahill, who used to run the Joslin Diabetes Center down here in Boston. He and I would talk for hours and hours, with Bud Veatch at the NIH, about how long people can go without food... this transition over from therapeutic fasting into starvation.

Also, it's like anything: Your body gets accustomed. You can go a long time without eating, if you're in shape. If you've done this. But it depends on what your body weight is, how old you are, it depends on a lot of different things. How long you can go without eating.

But the bottom line is: We were trying to develop a therapy and figure out the mechanisms by which ketogenic diets were therapeutic.

Dr. Attia:
Now, going back to the Cahill stuff for a moment, before we come back to that.

Did you have a sense, or did George have a sense of when those patients were in a negative nitrogen balance? And I assume it matters as to what their starting weight is and muscle mass, things like that. But were there general rules, about once you cross over that point, where you're basically pulling nitrogen out of the muscle?

Prof. Seyfried:
Right, right. He got that data actually from the 10 guys that starved to death in Mays Prison in Northern Ireland. He was there, monitoring their blood work. Dying of starvation...

Dr. Attia:
...these were prisoners, they were fasting as a protest?
(...)

Yes. It was pretty horrific. Now, those guys were all young Irishman in their 20s and 30s. I don't know what the oldest guy was. But they lived from, I don't know, 68 to 85, 90 days. Without any food, just water.

But then he subsequently fasted these very obese people...

Dr. Attia:
...for 40 days.

Prof. Seyfried:
Longer, for 6 months, 8 months.

Dr. Attia:
Oh, wow!

Prof. Seyfried:
Yeah, he has the data. One guy, a postman, lost his job. He weighed 450 pounds or something, couldn't deliver the mail anymore. So they put him on the water only fasting for 6 or 8 months. The guy lost 250 pounds.

Dr. Attia:
This is different from the other guy, right? There was a single case report of a patient who weighed a little over 400 pounds and did a 382 day fast.

Prof. Seyfried:
Yeah, I don't know if that was Cahill there. But he showed us the data on this one guy, the postman. And the issue of course is vitamins and minerals. I don't know if he took many supplements because bodyfat holds a lot of vitamins, fat soluble vitamins.

The minerals come from your bones. The liver control holds an awful lot of B vitamins and things like this. I think there were supplements over the course of the fast. You don't you need a lot of supplements, your body holds the things you need.

We evolved as a species to starve. I mean, our existence today is dependent on our ability to go long periods of time without eating. Well, not anymore.

Dr. Attia:
Yeah, and it seems that our ability to access minerals and vitamins is highly dependent on our nutritional state. In other words, your need for those things tends to go up in a fed state. At least according to some research I've seen.

Prof. Seyfried:
Yeah, you're right. And our ancestors were hardened people, their bodies were already acclimated to a starvation mode. So they were very efficient in maintaining mineral and nutrient balances.

I think in our society today - and this is purely speculation - a lot of the foods are depleted in the nutrients that we would need. Therefore, some people are almost like in a starvation mode, as they're eating foods that have no nutritional value. Consequently, you store a lot of fat.

Because the body doesn't usually get rid of sugar. As I said, sugar is stored, it's not peed out, sugar unless you have type 1 diabetes or something. The body has all these filtration systems to keep carbs in - which is then transferred to fat and stored as fat. The fat is our energy to keep us alive when there's no food.

But all these ideas and things were developing when we were doing the epilepsy studies. Then it became clear that calorie restriction was a key mechanism by which the ketogenic diet was working.

And we have since then seen in numerous children with epilepsy, that breakthrough seizures will occur when blood sugar spikes.

Dr. Attia:
Define spike in that very specific case: How high does it need to be in milligrams per deciliter?

Prof. Seyfried:
For managing epilepsy, there's many cases where it just has to go a little bit above the baseline. So kids will have a very low 70, 65 milligrams per dekaliter, they'll grab a cupcake at a party or whatever, that spikes it up to 120 mg/dl - and then you'll get a breakthrough seizure.

Dr. Attia:

Do you believe that it is the absolute value, of 120 in that case? Or do you believe it's the delta, the meaning the rate of change of the glucose?

Prof. Seyfried:

We can't know that, it hasn't been done to investigate that detail. I just know this from the clinicians and the nurses who have told me all this information. And of course, when your child has a breakthrough seizure... nobody likes to see a kid seizing! I mean, it's very traumatic. It's not a pleasant thing.

Once they realized that the kids have to maintain their blood glucose very stable, the parents are very, very restrictive of their diet. Because they don't want to see their child seize.

When we do the same thing for cancer: The problem with cancer is you don't see a breakthrough seizure. You don't see a group of tumor cells starting to grow faster. You don't see the immediate effects. They are there but you just can't see them.

With epilepsy, you have a very visible, clear indication that something went wrong. And unvariably, there is a spike in glucose.

Now, what's very interesting in these kids: They could be maintained for months without a single seizure - and then, one drink of grape juice or whatever, boom! Breakthrough seizure within sometimes minutes from the time of ingestion.

They can flip back. But then they can also get back on track again. They don't have a large number of seizures, they can just get back on track. But it's a very sensitive system in our brain.

As John Freeman told me: „We don't understand that when some kids are maintained seizure free or minimal seizures for long periods of time on ketogenic diets, and then we remove the diet - they seem to be managed!"

In other words, they don't return to their multiple seizures that they would have had every day. So he doesn't know, if it was because the diet did something fundamental or they outgrew the seizure or a different reason. Again, these are areas in epilepsy that are under active investigation.

Dr. Attia:

It's interesting, it's almost like a reset. I mean, one of the things that impressed me about reading the case studies of these very, very long fasts is that in the reports that were published several years later, many of the subjects maintain their new weight reduced state.

Which is a bit counterintuitive, based on what we know today about traditional dieting approaches, where everybody will sort of return back to baseline.

So it begs a question: When you starve this person for 6 months, do they completely change the way they eat on the other side? Because of a behavioral shift? Or is it a physiologic shift? Meaning, their metabolism has been kind of fixed?

Prof. Seyfried:
Well, I think it's probably a combination of both. These are very complicated physiological processes. They call it the thrifty gene, that was a term. It's not one gene, it's like thrifty physiology.

If you do yo-yo dieting, you can be screwed up for a long period of time. Those things all have loose ends. There's nothing that we have found that is absolutely consistent in all patients all the time, when it comes to those kinds of things.

And that's why they're always interesting to talk about. Because someone always has a new idea about something, regarding diets.

I don't really dwell, engage in those kinds of things, as far as our research is concerned. We know about them, we talk about them, but that's it. None other than the calorie restriction that we introduced into the mice.

To go back to the story, back to cancer: Then when we found out that the calorie restriction and the ketogenic diets were working. So people say „Well, why don't you just do calorie restriction?"

We don't like the term restriction. The term... you already have a disease, now you even have to be restricted. So, a ketogenic diet takes the sting out of a therapeutic fast. And they can also replicate some of the same physiological changes.

The key is to lower the blood sugar and to elevate the ketones, and that's what ketogenic diets do for managing epilepsy, and they do the same thing for cancer.

The issue, of course, is we don't know the mechanism by which lowering glucose and elevating ketones is responsible for the management of the seizure.

This is under active investigation by a lot of labs, that actual mechanism. Is it the elevation of the ketones? Is it the reduction of the glucose? Or is it some combination of the two?

But for cancer, it becomes very clear. The mechanism of action is very clear, for how this kills cancer cells: It's based on Otto Warburg's theory.

So when we started to do this and realized that calorie restriction was shrinking these tumors down massively, based on the drug that I told you about - because it was working through calorie restriction. Then I said „How does calorie restriction stop tumors?"

Then we realized that it was lowering blood sugar. So we started measuring blood sugar in these calorie restricted mice, and measuring ketones - and we were seeing that we were getting these major shifts. Then it became clear: Who was the guy who did this,o r thought about it? It was Otto Warburg.

Now, he wasn't doing ketogenic diets. Had he done and known about that, I think he would have been able to crack this cancer thing far, far earlier. He didn't do ketogenic diets, he didn't know a thing about that.

Dr. Attia:
So let's back up for a moment for people. I think, most people listening probably know what the Warburg Effect is and who Warburg was. But maybe, just give us a moment of setting the stage for what his observation was, that now bears his name.

Prof. Seyfried:
Well, his interest was in biochemistry. He was a classical biochemist in his time. He began to look at the metabolism of tumors.

He made an observation - which was solidified - that cancer cells continued to do an ancient fermentation metabolism, even in the presence of oxygen.

The Pasteur effect, Louis Pasteur, with the yeast was, that yeast will ferment...

That organism evolved to be able to ferment, to get energy in the absence of oxygen. But as soon as oxygen came into the presence, they stopped fermenting and they immediately started respiring. They have a system that can do that.

So the Pasteur effect was basically the termination of fermentation in the presence of oxygen. That was the Pasteur

154

effect. And it was repeated in all these yeast strains. That was a fundamental biochemical advancement, so to say.

But Warburg recognized - he knew Pasteurs worked very well - and he said, „Geez, these cancer cells, man! They continue to throw out lactic acid, even in the presence of a 100% oxygen!"

He grew cancer cells in 100% oxygen - and they would still make lactic acid! Clearly, with these cells, the Pasteur effect wasn't working.

Dr. Attia:
I'll just interject for a moment to explain something to the reader.

You convert glucose to pyruvate in the cytoplasm. And that yields a couple of units of ATP.

Then you have sort of a choice of what you're going to do with that pyruvate. If your demand for ATP is incredibly quick and high - usually exceeding the capacity of oxygen to get into the cell - you'll make lactate.

But that's also relatively inefficient, meaning you don't get that much more ATP, I think you get another 2 molecules of ATP per unit of pyruvate. But at least you have the advantage of saying I'm not limited by oxygen.

Alternatively, if oxygen is plentiful, and more importantly: If the demand for ATP is not excessive, you can shuttle that pyruvate into acetyl-CoA in the mitochondria, and you can generate over 30 units of ATP.

So what you're saying is: There was an observation which said „Hey, if I put this cell in the presence of lots of oxygen, it really shouldn't make much lactate."

Prof. Seyfried:
Right. That's what you'll find when you take normal tissue like kidney slices, muscle or liver slices, you'd grow them in 100% oxygen and they'd produce minimal, barely detectable lactate. There's always some going to be produced in every tissue, basically. It's very minimal.

But the cancer cell continues to dump out massive amounts of lactic acid, even in the presence of 100% oxygen!

So Warburg saw this over and over again. It didn't make any difference whether it was a human tumor, a mouse tumor or a rat tumor, they were all doing the same kind of thing.

What he concluded from this was that their respiratory system was defective. Because, like you just said with pyruvate: That's the Embden Meyerhoff pathway, going from glucose to pyruvate. Pyruvate is the end of that.

So then the opportunity is that the pyruvate would enter into the mitochondrial oxygenating conditions, and be fully oxidized to water and CO_2. Oxygen is the acceptor of the electrons, to form the water. And the carbons are coming from the foods that we metabolize.

But the cancer cell was dumping out large amounts of this lactic acid. Why would a cancer cell dump out lactic acid? It became clear to Warburg, through a variety of experiments, that the respiratory system was defective in these cells.

Dr. Attia:

Let's just clarify that: Many people, when they hear respiratory system, they think of lungs. What you really mean is the mitochondrial machinery that undergoes what we call cellular respiration.

Prof. Seyfried:

The lungs are bringing in the oxygen and getting rid of the CO_2. That enables the cells in our body to perform this very efficient form of energy production. Which then frees up the cells to do their sophisticated behaviors.

Liver cells do what they do, kidney cells, brain cells. They all do what they do because they have this very efficient energetic system. That's working because of this cellular mechanism called respiration.

The lungs are just the facilitators of the body to get the good air in and the bad air out.

So basically: The cancer cell was continuing to produce massive amounts of lactic acid, despite the fact that there was all this oxygen, this O_2. He was then looking at the mitochondria, noticing that there were some defects.

But he wasn't at the level of electron microscopy.

Dr. Attia:

What year? This is in the 1920s?

Prof. Seyfried:

Mostly late 20s, 30s, 40s. All the way up to the 50s. I think he stopped his research maybe in the early 60s.

Dr. Attia:

156

Now, he won a Nobel Prize, didn't he?

Prof. Seyfried:
Yes, he did.

Dr. Attia:
Was this for the description of this phenomenon?

Prof. Seyfried:
No, it was for the discovery of cytochrome c oxidase, which is actually one of the key enzymes in the electron transport chain. How cells generate energy through respiration.

He was nominated other times. And there's still some controversy about how many times he had been nominated for the work on cancer, but never to achieve another Nobel Prize.

He was considered one of the dominant biochemists in the 20th century. And he had very strong ideas and very excellent quantitative measurements for this, a lot of his work was reproduced by dozens and dozens of scientists.

So that was the fundamental observation. Then he extended this to this theory, regarding the question why are the cells are producing all this lactic acid? Because the organelle that is supposed to be involved is defective!

This led to a lot of controversy: „What do you mean, defective? How? What do you mean?"

Much later, Pete Peterson from John Hopkins did a magnificent job in collecting all this information. Peterson found that in every kind of a cancer cell - no matter what kind it is - there was some defect in the number, structure or function of the mitochondria. And it could vary.

- Some cancer cells have very few mitochondria but they look normal.
- Other tumor cells clearly have a lot of mitochondria, but they look abnormal.
- Whatever it was, it was something to do with an impairment of the respiratory system within the cell.

And if the cell can't generate energy through normal respiration, then it has to ferment There's no other way, they can't get the needed energy any other way.

One of the biggest problems in this whole thing is that the Warburg Effect is a secondary problem, that's subjected to many variants in the environment. But everybody focuses on this. The fermentation, the Warburg Effect, is not the issue.

The real issue is the damage to their respiration! And everybody says „No, respiration is normal in cancer cells." Why would they say it's normal?

Because they started doing cells in culture, rather than looking at the tissues themselves. Once you start doing culture work, you're taking cells from a tissue, separating them and growing them as if they were microorganisms in a culture dish.

Well, this changes everything. They're no longer connected to each other, they're growing in some artificial fluid, and they're doing things that they sometimes do and sometimes not do in the real world.

So you make a lot of assumptions about things, based on a system that itself is artificial.

Dr. Attia:
Let me ask a couple of technical questions:

Obviously, measuring the amount of lactate, or hydrogen ions that's produced, is a way to give us an indication of how much anaerobic metabolism is taking place. If you're not in cell culture, how do you quantify the amount of aerobic respiration?

Prof. Seyfried:
You look at the amount of oxygen consumed and the amount of lactic acid produced. So if you're doing aerobic respiration, you're consuming a lot of oxygen and producing very little lactate.

Then you can quantitate the amount of ATP being produced per milliliter of oxygen that you consume. This can vary anywhere from 7 ATP units to 9, depending on the system. Warburg used the number 7 based on his data at that time. So you could calculate the total amount of ATP being produced in the cell, based on its oxygen consumption and its lactic acid production.

Dr. Attia:
And Warburg did this in situ?

Prof. Seyfried:
Yes, he did it in slices and then he did it in cell culture as well. But with this, he created some of his own problems as well, switching from one to the other.

The concern that we have now is that many cells in culture look like they're consuming a lot of oxygen. And they're making lactic acid. But they're also consuming a lot of oxygen.

Dr. Attia:
So you're suggesting that they're doing both... which is still a bit odd.

Prof. Seyfried:
Yeah, right. Well, that was Sidney Winehouses argument:

His argument was the cancer cell needs so much energy that respiration by itself can't be sufficient. So they have to ferment and respire at the same time - and that made everybody feel that „Yeah, Warburg was wrong! They do have good respiration, but they just need so much more energy. They need to ferment at the same time."

But the work from Pete Peterson showed that they have defective respiration. I mean, they have defective mitochondria. Structure, number and function.

Besides, many other studies have shown that, too. They can't be doing oxidative phosphorylation or respiration, because the very organelle that is needed for that is deffective in some way.

And that could be in many different ways, as I said. All cancer cells have a defect in respiration. How that defect came about and how it manifests can vary from one type of cancer to another. One has to recognize that.

Not every cancer cell will have the exact same defect in respiration, in the mitochondria. Some will have very few mitochondria. So they just don't have quantitatively enough organelles to do respiration.

But what seems to be there, seems to be functional. Partially functional. Other cells, as I said, are loaded with mitochondria - but when you look at them, they're morphologically abnormal.

Structure dictates function! In biology, we know that structure dictates function. So if the structure of the organelle is abnormal, you know that the function of that organelle is not going to be normal.

Dr. Attia:
And is the idea that those those mutations were acquired?

Prof. Seyfried:
I wouldn't call them mutations, I would call them defects.

Dr. Attia:

In other words, the genome is unaffected in some of those cases?
Prof. Seyfried:
Yes, we've done that. We sequenced the entire genome of 5 different independently derived cancers, from mice. All derived from different origins - and we didn't find a single genetic abnormality! What we call pathogenic, where the mutation would actually have an effect on aunction. We didn't find a single one!
Dr. Attia:
Let's maybe take a step back. Because I think that for many people, there's an understanding that...

I mean, by definition, a cancer has a mutation that renders it incapable of listening to normal cell signaling.

Do you have a sense, broadly, of what amount of human cancers arise from germline mutations, rather than somatic mutations? It's obviously very small, but I don't know what the number is.
Prof. Seyfried:
Well, they say it's about 5-6%. You know, you hear about them. The BRCA1, P53...
Dr. Attia:
...Lynch syndrome, etc.
Prof. Seyfried:
Yeah. But when we looked into those... we call them inherited risk factors: None of them have ever been 100% penetrant! Which means that every person having that gene must not necessarily...
Dr. Attia:
...they are not purely deterministic.
Prof. Seyfried:
Yes. They're not deterministic. And as Warburg said, there are many secondary causes of cancer - but there's only one primary cause: The primary cause is the damage to the respiratory system.

So if the inherited mutation damages the respiratory system of the cell, then the probability of cancer is a real possibility. Because everybody who has Li-Fraumeni tumors or BRCA1 tumors or whatever, they're all fermenters.

The fermentation metabolism is there. In every cancer. But there are some people that have the exact same mutation that the other person has, but they never develop a tumor! Because,
160

for whatever reason, in that person that mutation did not damage the respiration.

Now, that could be an environmental suppressive effect, or another gene in the genome that prevents the inherited mutation from damaging the respiration. We don't know that. We only know that you don't get cancer if your mitochondria remain healthy. That's what we know.

That's important, because that goes back to the prevention issue, how do you prevent cancer? You prevent cancer by keeping your mitochondria healthy. How do you do that?

Well you avoid, if you can avoid, those risk factors. Mostly from the environment, like

- Viral infections
- Intermittent hypoxia
- Radiation exposure
- Carcinogenic exposure

All these different things. Every one of those things can damage respiration in a population of cells, then leading to cancer. Because we know of no cancer that has normal respiration.

So when you grow them in culture, people say „Yeah, they have normal respiration! They are taking in oxygen, so therefore Warburg is wrong."

But when you look at the structure in vivo, you look at the tissues and you look at the actual architecture of the tissue, invariably you find damage to the respiration. Damage to the structure and function of these mitochondria.

So what the field has done is: They've put more credibility into the results from cell culture work, than studies that use the actual tissues from patients or rodents.

Dr. Attia:
The Warburg Effect was largely forgotten for many years, after his initial observation. Right?

Prof. Seyfried:
Yeah, a lot of what he did was forgotten, Pete Peterson was one of the few guys that kept the fire burning. As I said: When Watson and Crick discovered the DNA, the origin of the genetic material... it wasn't only them, there was a whole group of other

people that were doing it, they just weren't acknowledged as much.

After the discovery of the DNA, the field ran off into that. They knew that there were chromosomal abnormalities in some cancer, so it made clear that „Hey, you know: These genomic defects in the tumor cells are likely the real origin of the disease!"

So the whole field more or less shifted away from the traditional biochemical analysis to this more molecular biology analysis. Therefore, you find more and more mutations, more and more genetic defects and all these kinds of things, leading people to believe that these were the causes of the disease.

A lot of really nice experiments were done, where they would introduce mutant virus particles into cells, and they would integrate into the nuclear genome. Then you'd see that the cancer cells become transformed into a neoplastic kind of a cell, giving the appearance that this was a causal effect.

They didn't realize that those same viruses went into the mitochondria and blew out the respiration! That wasn't even considered as possible.

Dr. Attia:

If the viruses are doing that, presumably, they're integrating into the genome?

Prof. Seyfried:

Yeah, they would do it both ways. Viruses can do it in a lot of different ways. So sometimes the viruses actually infect directly into the mitochondria. They produce proteins in the mitochondria that screw up the electron transport chain.

Other times, the viruses integrate into the nuclear genome, producing a protein product that then disrupts the mitochondria.

Either way, the mitochondria are disrupted! Whether it's
- a direct effect, the virus replicating inside the organelle. Or
- it's an effect of a product produced by the virus, that then goes and disrupts the organelle.

This is what we're finding for the majority of these situations. So even the inherited mutations that we look at, they disrupt mitochondrial function. And if they disrupt mitochondrial function, you are at risk for developing a neoplasm in that particular population of cells.

Dr. Attia:
There are some cancers that don't follow that, correct? I mean, aren't there some cancers that have normal mitochondria?

Prof. Seyfried:
We haven't found any. The evidence for that is that they're all fermenting. We haven't found a cancer that doesn't ferment. So if the cancer is fermenting, it's obviously not respiring. If its respiration would be normal, it shouldn't be fermenting.

As a matter of fact, Dean Burke did this kind of a study, way back in the 50s. He looked at various kinds of hepatomas. Because there was an article, saying there was this very slow growing hepatoma that did not ferment.

But Burke - who was the head of the NCI at the time - studied these things in massive detail. He was able to show that the slowest growing tumor did have a significant elevation of lactic acid production over a normal cell - but you had to look at it really carefully and do the experiments over extended periods of time.

So even the slowest of the slowest growing tumors, guys that maybe would be considered benign, were still making lactic acid.

Another interesting thing is the crown gall tumors in plants: Plants have cancer, but they don't metastasize. They just grow, these tumors.

And people back in the 30s were testing Warburg's theory in these plants. And: They all had damaged respiration! They were fermenting, just like the mouse tumors.

Dr. Attia:
When you say respiration, you mean photosynthetic respiration?

Prof. Seyfried:
No, plants have both. Plants can get energy from chloroplasts to build carbohydrates, but they also have mitochondria.

Dr. Attia:
I didn't realize that. So their carbon fixation obviously comes from photosynthesis. But when they make their equivalent of starch...

Prof. Seyfried:
...yes, they will burn their owns fuels to generate respiratory energy. But they also have dysmorphic cell growth, and they've

called these crown gall tumors. You see them sometimes on the side of trees.

So people back in the day analyzed the biochemistry of these things, and they also found that they were following Warburg's metabolic profile. But they didn't metastasize.

The reason they don't metastasize is: They don't have an immune system. It turned out, from our work and the work of others, that the metastatic cell is actually part of our immune system!

So macrophages and leukocytes, these are the cells that have the genetic capability of moving around the body, entering into tissues. This is what they do.

Plants don't have that. Plants don't have that kind of an immune system. So the cancers in plants don't metastasize, they grow in place. But humans, and other animals of course, have these cells of the immune system. Therefore they can get metastatic cancer.

Dr. Attia:
Before we get to that:

Another argument that's been proposed for the Warburg Effect is the need for cellular building blocks. The thing that the tumor specfically is doing is growing, although not necessarily faster than a regular cell.

It certainly grows in a less regulated way and therefore it's going to proliferate. Matthew Vander Heiden, Lewis Cantley and Craig Thompson wrote that paper in 2009, I'm sure you're familiar with. That was a Science paper, I believe.

And they proposed this other explanation, which was: „Look, it's not just an energetic thing!" In fact, I don't recall if they said „It's not just-„ or „It's not even about the energetics."

But the point here was... this is where you get building blocks to make cells grow. Do you think it's possible that both of these are correct?

Prof. Seyfried:
Well, in the process of upregulating the Emden-Meyerhoff pathway, you are gonna get the carbons for building blocks. At the same time, you're going to get some energy. Through the pyruvate kinase system.

However, very interesting: They deviate from the path from Warburg's theory, in saying that respiration is normal. Okay?

164

They think there's nothing wrong with the mitochondria. They've said that many times, Craig Thompson has said this.

You have to ignore a massive amount of evidence to make those kinds of statements. You just have to ignore everything that Pete Peterson has done. Which is a life's work, showing that the mitochondria have abnormalities.

Thompson doesn't even mention that, they don't discuss Pete Peterson's massive amount of evidence.

But you're right: In order for a cell to grow, you need a lot of building blocks. And you need carbon. Where's the carbon coming from? It's coming from both the pentose pathway and the glycolytic pathway, and it's also coming from glutamine.

These cancer cells are sucking down glutamine. So you're getting the amide nitrogen to form the nucleotides, you're getting the glutamate, that then goes into anaplerosis in the TCA cycle.

So between glucose and glutamine, you aren't getting all of the building blocks that you need for rapid cell division. But where is the energy coming from? Without energy, nothing grows! Nothing can live without ATP. So where is the energy coming from?

This is our thing. So we, Christos Chinopoulos in Hungary and I, proposed this a long time ago, on a purely theoretical basis. Having been convinced that Warburg was right - that the respiration of all cancer cells is damaged to some extent.

So if that's the case, the Warburg Effect was only the glucose part of the puzzle. It wasn't the glutamine part of the puzzle.

Now with our new information, we know that most of the ATP in the cancer is coming from substrate level phosphorylation in the mitochondria (SLP=fermenting), which is disconnected from oxidative phosphorylation (OxPhos=Breathing, respiratory)

What we have now is the missing link in Warburg's basic theory.

Dr. Attia:
Explain what substrate level phosphorylation, what SLP is.

Prof. Seyfried:
Substrate level phosphorylation is the production of ATP, when you move a phosphate group from an organic substrate onto an ADP molecule. It's an ancient way of generating energy.

In other words: It's an organic molecule that's an electron acceptor, rather than oxygen.

Dr. Attia:

Right. Instead of going through the electron transport chain, where you use NAD, NADH and ADP, NADPH as electron transporters...

Prof. Seyfried:

...well, electron donors...

Dr. Attia:

Eletron donors, you can do a very quick trick where you take an ADP, meaning it has two phosphates, and restore it. You restore it to an ATP by using an organic molecule that donates a phosphate.

Prof. Seyfried:

For substrate level phosphorylation, yes. So succinyl-CoA has a phosphate group, and that phosphate group is then donated to ADP - sometimes GDP to make GTP, depends on the situation.

But in cancer cells, it's ATP. So you're moving phosphate groups from an organic substrate onto the ADP as the acceptor. And you can generate massive amounts of energy from that process. Which can replaces the level of lost energy from oxidative phosphorylation.

Dr. Attia:

And does that occur inside the mitochondria? Inside the inner matrix?

Prof. Seyfried:

Yes, it's in the matrix. So you're gonna make a lot of ATP. It's gonna just replace it.

- In the normal cell, you're making most of the ATP from oxidative phosphorylation.
- In the cancer cell, you're making most of it from substrate level phosphorylation.

Inside the same organelle.

Dr. Attia:

Why don't our cells do this under demand? So if we jumped up and down and did 25 burpees right now, we would very quickly exceed our oxidative capacity for respiration. And we'd start making a bunch of lactate. Why aren't we also undergoing SLP?

Prof. Seyfried:
Well, we do, in the heart muscles. They've done various cardiac and restriction experiments and things like that. A lot of this has been worked down in the heart, so it does happen. We do do substrate level phosphorylation, but it only can be done for short periods of time. It can't be done extensively.

You can't replace oxidative phosphorylation - under normal conditions - with substrate level phosphorylation. When you hold your breath, you're only gonne be able to survive for a certain period of time. The lacitic acid builds up too much.

I mean, this was shown by Jose Kozka, when he did some incredibly interesting experiments, trying to hold various aquatic animals under water and looking at the metabolic changes that occurred. Seals, porpoises, turtles and all these kinds of things.

He strapped them to a board, held them under water - and then he would measure all these metabolites in the bloodstream.

Now, these were animals that actually could live under water. If that would be done to humans, we'd all be dead. We couldn't live that long, but 5 minutes at the most. But these animals could live 10, 15, 20 minutes being held under water. And they weren't breathing, of course.

Now, they were stressed out because they were strapped to a board. But the bottom line is: He started measuring all these metabolites in the bloodstream. Lactic acid goes right up in massive amounts. You'd expect that.

Succinic acid is another interesting thing. So succinic acid, in the TCA cycle, is a powerful stimulatory towards oxidative phosphorylation. And it was being dumped out into the circulation. Meaning, it wasn't being oxidized.

He claimed that it was amino acid fermentation that was doing this. So the body was grabbing amino acids, metabolizing them and generating energy through substrate level phosphorylation.

Well, it turns out: The cancer cell is doing this in a massive amount, because they don't have the OxPhos. You look at cancer cells and they're dumping out succinic acid. And succinic acid stabilizes 1α. So you can continue to increase the transcription factors that are driving fermentation.

This whole thing is just a massive shift from OxPhos to substrate level phosphorylation.

Dr. Attia:
Does creatinephosphate fit into that SLP pathway, or is that totally separate?

Prof. Seyfried:
I'm not sure about that. It could be a source of the phosphate groups, but I haven't looked into that. Dominic may know a lot more about that than I do.

Dr. Attia:
So when you go back to... there's an undercurrent here, to what we're talking about. Which is: The view that you hold is the minority view today. It sounds like.

Prof. Seyfried:
It's just a matter of time.

Dr. Attia:
Why do you think that is? What do you think is the...

I mean, I know people want to come up with conspiracy theories. That's one of the things about social media that I find frustrating, is, people always want a conspiracy theory to be the explanation.

Like „Oh, the drug companies don't want this to be true" or something. I find those things hard to believe.

Do you think there's a better explanation for why these hypotheses are not being investigated, with the rigor they should be?

Prof. Seyfried:
Well, you have to look at the discipline of the individuals that are working on the project. Okay? Most of the people doing cancer research are molecular biologists. Being a molecular biologist, you have a certain perspective on the nature of the problem.

You don't look at respiration directly. You look at gene expression profiles that may be directly or indirectly related to that. And then you make claims about what's going on.

So most of the people are of a discipline that says that genes are changed - they are not looking at the actual consumption of oxygen and production of lactic acid, not looking at what Warburg actually looked at. Then you have a very different explanation for what's happening.

A lot of people today use the seahorse instrument to measure oxygen consumption. When you put cancer cells and tumor cells, normal cells, into a dish, they're all taking up oxygen similarly - and therefore Warburg must be wrong.

Warburg also said that both tumor cells and normal cells will take up oxygen at the same rate. Except the tumor cell is uncoupled and the normal cell is not uncoupled - which means that the oxygen uptake in the tumor cell is not linked directly to ATP production. People ignore that!

Dr. Attia:
How would one measure that? ATP is very tricky to measure, ATP production.

Prof. Seyfried:
ATP can be measured. The problem is what's the origin of it?

Dr. Attia:
That's what I mean, it's tricky to isolate the ATP source. Let's say you have a tumor cell and a non tumor cell, and they're both taking up lots of oxygen as measured by calorimetry and one's producing a bunch of lactate.

But how can you tell if the cancer cell is taking up oxygen and not making ATP?

Prof. Seyfried:
If it's taking up oxygen... well, if it doesn't make ATP, it's dead. Right?

Dr. Attia:
Sorry: If it's not making the ATP commensurate with its oxygen consumption.

Prof. Seyfried:
Well, sometimes you look at that and you'd say „Wow, look at the oxygen consumption! Is the ATP production commensurate with oxygen uptake?"

Dr. Attia:
Yes. That would be coupled. Wouldn't it?

Prof. Seyfried:
As long as it's not producing lactic acid or succinic acid.

Dr. Attia:
I'm a bit confused, why couldn't it do both?

Couldn't a cell undergo anaerobic metabolism, make ATP that is accounted for by the amount of lactate that's produced - but similarly take up oxygen, and in a coupled fashion, make ATP there?

Prof. Seyfried:

That's an important point, because a lot of people stumble on that. The problem is:

When you're looking at the ATP production coming out of the mitochondria, it's not always easy to know whether it's generated by a coupled mechanism (where the oxygen is in fact linked to the ATP through FoF1-ATPase) or whether it's coming from mitochondria substrate level phosphorylation.

Dr. Attia:

Ah, got it. It's not easy to do the mass balance of this many mols of oxygen were produced (or consumed) and this many mols of ATP were produced. You can't do that math, do you?

Prof. Seyfried:

Yeah... well, Warburg did that, but he was looking...

Dr. Attia:

He didn't know about SLP, right?

Prof. Seyfried:

Well, lactic acid production... The production of ATP, the pyruvate kinase, is substrate level phosphorylation. But it's cytoplasmic.

Dr. Attia:

Yes, yes, it's not mitochondrial.

Prof. Seyfried:

No, he did not know. He couldn't have known because the very systems, they didn't come out until the 50s, 60s. Of which we know now that there is another form of ATP production inside the mitochondria.

What people have failed to realize is: Every biochemical textbook says we only get 2% oxygen coming out of the mitochondria, through substrate level phosphorylation. Just like we get from the cytoplasm.

But for cancer cells, people say „Oh, you can get a lot more ATP from the cytoplasm." Not thinking that you can upregulate the same phenomenon inside the mitochondria! As a matter of fact, we think that substrate level phosphorylation in the mitochondria is far greater than the amount of ATP produced in the cytoplasm.

A number of people have found that the PKM2 isoform of pyruvate kinase doesn't make much ATP. It makes a buttload of lactic acid, but it's not linked to the ATP production! So therefore they have to say „Respiration is normal", because the cell is making so much ATP.

But if Otto Warburg is correct, and all of the structural biochemistry is correct, the mitochondria can't be making ATP from OxPhos. It can't be, because the structure of the organelle is defective. So where the hell is all that damn ATP coming from inside that organelle?

And then when you look at the data that we have... and glutamine is being consumed in massive amounts. So it's got to be coming from substrate level phosphorylation.

Dr. Attia:
What is the fundamental structural defect in the mitochondria? Which is interesting, I'd never thought until this discussion about the possibility that you could have a completely normal mitochondrial genome and just have structural defects.

Then obviously, you can have genetic abnormalities that lead to protein productions that create structual problems.

But in the former case, having a perfectly normal mitochondrial genome, but now you have a defect: What is the actual physical defect?

Prof. Seyfried:
In the number, in the structure? It can happen in many different ways.

For example, if a carcinogen enters into the mitochondria, they cause a lot of oxidative stress. What we found in our massive studies... this is how we got onto knowing that Otto Warburg was in fact correct.

I mean, at first I didn't know what the hell was going on, like like everybody else. But when we found no mutations in the mitochondrial DNA and we knew these cells were fermenting, because they were making a lot of lactic acid - then we started looking at the lipids inside the mitochondrial lipidome. We call it the lipidome.

We found that cardiolipin, the signature lipid in the inner membrane, is defective in all the tumor cells that we've ever looked at!

That tells us right there, that there's a problem in the function. Then we linked that to abnormalities in OxPhos.

171

So clearly, if the lipids are abnormal, that would affect the function of the proteins of the electron transport chain. Therefore you're not going to generate the amount of ATP through oxidative phosphorylation. Because the very lipid- and protein structures are abnormal. You just can't produce the amount of ATP.

That's supports Warburg, he knew that there were many problems within the mitochondrial function, that would then force the cell into fermentation. So what did they ferment? They ferment lactic acid and succinic acid.

What are the fuels for that? It's glucose and glutamine. So glucose and glutamine are ultimately the fuels that drive the cancer. They drive it through a process of substrate level phosphorylation. Occurring in the cytoplasm, where they can build a lot of metabolites for growth.

Also through the pathway called glutaminolysis.

Dr. Attia:

Now, one can't render glucose zero – meaning there's no dietary or pharmacologic intervention that could reduce glucose levels to zero. Are there any that could do that with glutamine?

Prof. Seyfried:

Let me just address the glucose issue: We can't get to zero, but we can get damn close to it! Alright? We have people in published papers, people who are on powerful therapeutic water, fasting only - and then given large injections of insulin...

Dr. Attia:

Sure, and they get to below 1 millimolar of blool glucose

Prof. Seyfried:

Yeah, even 0.5! (Laughter)

Dr. Attia:

Ha! But sustainably, it's very difficult to be below about 3 millimolar. Right?

Prof. Seyfried:

Right, right. But here's the situation:

The problem is when you do that, when you're going into calorie restriction. Restrictive ketogenic diets - you already are lowering the blood sugar to a significant degree. And what we found is that glucose transporters actually get upregulated in the normal cells, when you start doing this.

So the normal cells become glucose hungry and they become direct competitors now with the tumor cells. Those tumor cells absolutely need the glucose because the normal cells can burn the ketones and stay alive, the tumor cells can't burn the ketones - as their mitochondria are defective.

You need a good mitochondrial system to burn ketones for energy! So what we do, by calorie restriction and restricted ketogenic diets, is:

We make the normal cells glucose hungry and we transition them over to ketones. Keeping them alive, but they're still glucose hungry - and they are now competing directly with the tumor cells that absolutely have to have the glucose.

(...)

Our goal is to emerge from the therapy healthier than when you started it. So the question becomes:

How low can you get blood sugar without compromising the health status of the individual? Again, if you're in ketosis, you can push your blood sugars down really low.

Dr. Attia:

But you want to do this without insulin because insulin itself is protumorigenic, isn't it?

Prof. Seyfried:

Only if the blood sugars are high enough. Once you get those blood sugars down and you take away all the glucose from the body, or the majority of it, it kills the tumor cells. We have the data to support that.

(...)

Dr. Attia:

You're saying insulin does not function as a growth signal, outside of its anabolic activity in taking up glucose?

Prof. Seyfried:

Well, if you have high insulin-like growth factor, that is linked to the insulin of course That facilitates the uptake of glucose. I meant in general: If you don't have glucose, what else is going on? Because without ATP, you can't get energy anyway.

So our goal is to deplete the sources of fuel to the cells. So insulin, you can't eat insulin. Now, insulin drives the pyruvate dehydrogenase complex, which facilitates cancer growth.

That's why they say Oh, you can get this and that. But, that's only if you have a lot of glucose around, then insulin becomes

173

tumorigenic. But if you have very little glucose and you give more insulin, remove it, then it doesn't stimulate tumor growth. We have direct evidence to support that.

In fact, the Germans used to do that. They used to put people into insulin comas. The problem is, you don't want anybody to go into an insulin coma! If they were in ketosis, you could give it a sh*tload of insulin and they're not gonna die. We already have evidence in the literature to support that.

So you got to keep the door shut on that glucose as tight as you can, without harming the rest of the body. We use insulin, and then we do hyperbaric chambers - but that comes only after you shut the door on glucose and glutamine.

Dr. Attia:
How do you shut the door on glutamine?

Prof. Seyfried:
For the glutamine door, you have to use drugs. And the best drug we found so far is DON 6-diazo-5-oxo-L-norleucin. It's an old drug, was made years ago.

They used to use it on cancer patients, but they never targeted glucose at the same time. So the tumor cells were sucking down the glucose.

As a matter of fact, you can even make them more glucose sensitive if you take away the glutamine.

Dr. Attia:
So there's no dietary strategy that could effectively reduce glutamine?

Prof. Seyfried:
No, glutamine is a non-essential amino acid, we make it ourselves. We can even make glutamine from glucose. That's why it's called non-essential.

However, in physiology terms it is essential. It plays a massive role in the gut, in the immune system and in the urea cycle.

It's such an important amino acid, it's ubiquitous. It's the most abundant amino acid in our body!

Dr. Attia:
Yeah, that's a funny distinction. I'm glad you pointed that out. I'm sure that there are people listening to this who get confused by the term essential and non-essential regarding amino acids. It's 8 of them are essential in 12 are not essential, or something to that effect.

But what you're pointing out is an important distinction: They're non-essential because we don't have to get them exogenously. But: They are still essential for our survival, once produced endogenously.

Prof. Seyfried:
Yes, absolutely. Glutamine, it's the most abundant amino acid in our serum. It's everywhere. And our immune system...

Dr. Attia:
The point being, there's nothing you're gonna eat or not eat, that's gonna change that, right?

Prof. Seyfried:
No, people ask me that all the time. Changing your blood serum glutamine by eating differently is not possible. You got to do it with a drug but it has to be done strategically! You have to have people that are knowledgeable about this. You can't just have some guy just jack you up with a drug that blocks glutamine.

Because your immune system will be compromised - and our immune system is needed for the health of our gut, killing bacteria. And if you paralyze it too much, then you're going to get infections. You're going to have all kinds of other issues.

That's why we developed the press-pulse concept: You press the glucose hard with diets and drugs, and then you pulse the glutamine. What we think is going to happen is:

We will target the glutamine with a drug that will selectively kill tumor cells, by doing that we paralyze the immune system - but then immediately, we give large amounts of glutamine back. The drug is pulsed only.

The benefit of course is that you're going to restore your gut, you're going to restore your immune system - they're only paralyzed, they're not killed.

Dr. Attia:
When you say immune system, are you referring to the cellular or humoral system?

Prof. Seyfried:
Cellular, mostly.

Dr. Attia:
Because you've kind of implicated the humoral system, with the macrophage. In terms of mutagenesis.

Prof. Seyfried:
Well, we're talking about the cellular immune system

Dr. Attia:
Yes, you're talking about the T cells...
Prof. Seyfried:
...and B cells and macrophages. And natural killer cells, leukocytes, all these kinds of things. They're all heavily glutamine dependent. Okay?

So if you have a patient that has skinburns, opened up to bacteria, you have to give large amounts of glutamine because the immune system is needed to kill the bacteria.

You have to restore the gut function. A lot of the cells in the gut are glutamine dependent. So that's why you give a large amounts of glutamine to cancer patients, that have been burned.

But the problem is, of course, the tumor cells are using the same fuel. And: If you kill too many of the tumor cells too quickly, you've got to have a cell system to remove the corpses.

That's what the macrophages do and some of these other immune cells. They'll come in and remove the corpses, the dead cells. Otherwise you get infections, you die from the indirect effects of these things. So you have to know how to strategically target glutamine, without compromising the normal physiological systems that we have.

Dr. Attia:
Before we get into the therapeutic stuff, which I understand is probably what everybody wants to hear about...

I still want to get back to understanding some of this stuff a little bit better.

Experimentally, I'm still struggling with this chasm in belief systems, between what sounds like the majority of people who take the view that says:

Look, the respiratory system of the cancer cell is relatively normal. If you're seeing an increase in fermentation, it's an artifact of a higher throughput of substrate to generate more building blocks.

This strikes me as a very testable hypothesis, this really shouldn't be... we shouldn't be debating this! There should be a set of experiments that could resolve that.

Prof. Seyfried:
Yes, I think that diagram there on the board is the illustration of the strategy to test that hypothesis, basically. Which is:

The bottom line is: Where are they getting their energy from? If you stop their energy flow...

Dr. Attia:

The board picture we're talking about here is basically the TCA cycle, along with everything outside of the TCA cycle as well. There's even metabolic pathways that I can't name at this moment.

Prof. Seyfried:

You have to try to integrate. Like you said, you have to try to integrate all of the knowledge that we have on the biochemical systems into a strategy to manage the disease. And I break it down into some more simplistic things. In other words, energy. Without energy nothing grows.

The evidence that I'm convinced about, that I've read - massive amounts of literature - and looked carefully at everything, is:

The structure and function of the mitochondria in tumor cells is compromised. That's a fact! In my mind, that is a solid fact - and for somebody to deny that, one would have to ignore the evidence that I've looked at.

You have to look at mitochondria and say „No, that mitochondria that has no cristae and is very few in number, there's nothing wrong with it!" Okay? Let's call it black and white.

Dr. Attia:

Let's go one step further, because there is an objective way to assess structure... but shouldn't we just ask the functional question? Experimentally, I mean.

Prof. Seyfried:

Of course, and we do that. We know structure dictates function, that's a common in biology. Then, if that structure looks abnormal at the electron microscopy level, at various levels, why don't we look now at the activity of the proteins in the electron transport chain?

Dr. Attia:

This may be a naive question, but there can be large ranges of structure, that could still produce optimal function. And you would think that for something as important as respiration...

Which, to your point, might be the single most important function of a cell, as evidenced by the fact that toxins like cyanide are uniformly fatal within seconds.

...you'd think that the structural leeway within a mitochondria would be so high that you could...

Let's just say you could quantify structure as a scale from 1 to 10 - and obviously, a 10 out of 10 structure is perfectly functional. You'd want to believe that thing would function good enough, down to like a 2 out of 10. And only if you were staggeringly compromised everything go to hell.

So in other words, just to push back for a moment:

One could argue „Hey! Yeah, of course there's structural changes. But they're not functionally relevant because they're within a parameter space."

Prof. Seyfried:

Yes, that's an important point and I think the normal flexibility of our cells is able to accommodate those kinds of changes, over a short period of time. Mitochondria is such an incredibly vibrant system, it's a living organelle inside of ourselves.

It's a separate organism, actually.

Dr. Attia:

Separate DNA!

Prof. Seyfried:

Right. And they've turned over all of their DNA to the nucleus, except for 13 critical genes. Those 13 critical genes control the life of the cell!

Why should do this activity when I can get a dumb ass nucleus to do it for me? But I'm still gonna hold the keys to the kingdom.

There's still 13 genes, if anything goes wrong with them, you're dead.

This is the whole thing, why cancer cells don't die through the apoptotic mechanism. Because the very organelle that controls the kill switch, the switch doesn't work! So the cell bypasses the normal control of cell apoptosis (programmed cell death) in the cell, because the very organelle that dictates that is now defective!

Consequently, this cell now is reverting back to the way it existed before oxygen came into the atmosphere on the planet. They were all fermenters, they grew with unbridled proliferation, until the fermentable fuel in the environment was used up - and they all died.

So it was very clear what was going on before oxygen came into the atmosphere. Cells would proliferate unbridledly.

178

Albert Szent-Györgyi, his Alpha Period and the Existence of the Planet. So everything was working on substrate level phosphorylation. It was no oxidative phosphorylation. They were all doing that.

What we have in our system today are these same capabilities, but we don't use them. Only for very short periods of time, under various physical physiological stress situations. They don't become permanent.

In the cancer cell, they have become adapted. As Warburg said:

You can't get a cancer cell from a cell that cannot ferment.

So neurons in the brain can't ferment for very long. You rarely, if ever, get a tumor out of a neuron. Except neuroblastoma, which is outside the brain.

Heart cardiac myocytes rarely form cancers, even muscle cells rarely form cancers. Cells that need a of oxidative phosphorylation rarely can form a tumor. Only tumors can form in those cells that can upregulate fermentation pathways.

If you can't do that, you're gonna die.

Dr. Attia:

But wait, wouldn't skeletal muscle be one of the highest candidates to be able to upregulate fermentation, given their ATP demand?

Prof. Seyfried:

Yes, but they have a syncytium of mitochondria inside the muscles. They've adapted, this is part of their normal physiology. They can ferment for limited periods of time, under extreme stressful conditions. But: They can't permanently do that. They die.

The muscles will die on you, the cells will die if you try to force them into a long-term fermentation metabolism. But they have the capacity to operate fermentation for short periods of time, like many cells do.

But brain can't do that, heart can't do that.

Dr. Attia:

This is an interesting point you bring up. Let's go back to a myosite within my quadricep versus an epithelial cell in my colon.

To your point: The probability I will get a cancer that comes from the myosite in my quadricep is virtually zero?

179

Prof. Seyfried:
No, I didn't say virtually zero.
Dr. Attia:
I mean, outside of a sarcoma.
Prof. Seyfried:
Well, what's the origin of the sarcoma? What kind of cell?
Dr. Attia:
Depends, it can be a various kinds. But just for a moment, probability-wise, the myosite my quadriceps or my pecs, or something, forming cancer is so much lower than the epithelial cell in my colon, right?
Prof. Seyfried:
Yeah. Or an epithelial cell in your kidney, in the bladder, one of these kinds of things.
Dr. Attia:
I just picked colon because it's such a high cancer probability.
Prof. Seyfried:
Sure, breast is another one.
Dr. Attia:
Right. So explain to me again, the difference in their...

I would say like the muscle cell is far more adaptable at making lactate, when it needs to. Because I demand of it much more [lactate production during exercise] than I demand of my colonic epithelial cell.

But then... say what you were saying again, about the toxicity of lactate to that cell versus the epithelial cell in my colon.
Prof. Seyfried:
Well, the epithelial cell in your colon, it's a longer process. You don't go from a normal cell to a cancer cell over night, in a colon.

There are some situations where cancer can happen much quicker than people would normally think. But in general, it's a protracted process.

The cell has to have the capacity to shift from an oxidative process to a fermentation process. You have to have the machinery in the cell to be a fermenter because without that capacity you can never become a tumour cell.

Because cancer is a two-fold process:
1)   The gradual chronic interruption in respiratory function, coupled with

2) a gradual compensatory shift to the alternative form of energy, which is substrate level phosphorylation.

So if the cell is incapable of making that shift, it will never become a cancer cell. It can't, because in order to be a cancer cell, you have to be able to replace OxPhos with fermentation.

If you can't do that, you're not going to become a cancer cell. That's why brain neurons rarely become tumor cells, because they can't do that. Brain cells die.

If you interrupt oxidative phosphorylation in the neurons of our brain - we call that neuro-degeneration... So, we don't generally get tumors. We get tumors from the glial cells and the microglia, these kinds of things.

Dr. Attia:
I know what you're saying but maybe the reader will be confused by this. Because they're gonna say „But gosh, my aunt had brain cancer"...

It's very important that we distinguish between the glial cells and the neurons.

Prof. Seyfried:
Right, and the microglia.

Dr. Attia:
When we heat about astrocytomas - which would be the most common brain tumors - the cancer is not existing in the neuron.

Prof. Seyfried:
That's correct. Or cardiomyocytes, they just die. They are packed with mitochondria, but when they start fermenting, they die. They can't deal with that.

Dr. Attia:
Again. See, that's the part that just confuses me. It's so counterintuitive!

I would think that if there's gonna be a cell in my body that I want to be able to buffer lactate, specifically buffer the hydrogen ion that comes with it, that's actually what's killing this cell.

I would want my cardiac myocyte to be the single most robust cell in the body - because it has to be the last guy standing.

Prof. Seyfried:
Yeah. You know, this is the whole thing: When you get a heart attack, you die from brain damage. You don't die from the things people think you die of. Your liver and kidneys are fine.

That's why you can donate your liver and kidneys when you have a heart attack because those cells are not dying.

Dr. Attia:

Yeah, the brain is most susceptible to the hypoxia.

But the point is: Even at the level of the highest stress, I would want my cardiac myocytes to be able to access all fuels. Glucose, fatty acids, ketones.

Prof. Seyfried:

Well, they do that with degenerative heart disease, but they don't form cancer. They have a capacity... and this is where we found a lot of substrate level phosphorylation in the mitochondria. You see, the TCA cycle was discovered in stressed hearts!

Because they were saying that „The heart should be dead. Why is it still functioning here, where's the ATP coming from?"- and they found that most of the energy in the heart is coming from mitochondrial substrate level phosphorylation.

For shorter periods of time. Of course, you can't do this as a permanent shift. But the concepts were developed from the work in the heart. The same with the brain. I mean, if your brain is damaged, you can't function either.

So, the two organs, heart and brain, are remarkably dependent on oxidative phosphorylation for function. And disruptions of oxidative phosphorylation are usually catastrophic for those cells.

Dr. Attia:

I think I understand your argument, I was thinking about it in reverse.

You're saying because the brain and the cardiac myocytes have evolved to be so efficient under oxidative conditions, it's not so much that lactate is harmful to them. It's once that once you start to disrupt...

If the hypothesis is correct that it's the disruption in the mitochondria and its capacity to carry out OxPhos is the thing that's harmful, you die long before you bother getting cancer. Those cells undergo apoptosis or just die, right?

Prof. Seyfried:

Yes, yes, that's the point. The key is: How long does it take to transition a cell from an oxidative phosphorylation state into a cell that can become a tumor. Like in a colon cell as you mentioned.

Dr. Attia:
So the real problem that these other cells have, where cancer is so ubiquitous - whether it'd be breast or colon, according to this hypothesis - would be their metabolic flexibility. It's their capacity to easily wax and wane between...
I shouldn't say that, it's not their flexibility. It's their lack of dependency on oxidative phosphorylation.
Prof. Seyfried:
They depend... I mean, obviously like you said, with cyanide: It shuts it down and everything's dead real quick.
Dr. Attia:
If that happens so quickly that they don't have the ebb and flow.
Prof. Seyfried:
It's their capacity to upregulate fermentation over time, it doesn't happen overnight. It's a very gradual thing. Heart cardiomyocytes and neurons of the brain can't do that what these other cells are capable of doing.

What happens is this mitochondrial stress response - and this is where your oncogenes come in now. Because the oncogenes are transcription factors that upregulate fermentation pathways.

Basically, you when you damage the respiratory system of a cell, if 1α becomes stabilized, now you can upregulate glucose transporters into the cell. They all overlap each other. Lactic acid dehydrogenase...

In all these enzymes that are geared for maintaining a
fermentation metabolism,
the transcription factors that make those
pathways upregulated are the oncogenes, basically.

So the oncogenes have to facilitate... If you're not going to get the same level of energy out of your OxPhos, you've got to compensate. As I tell everybody:
The singular most largest consumer of energy in any cell is the pumps. These pumps that are on the surface of the cells that maintain the ionic gradients, that allow what we call life with it - because once you reach equilibrium, you're dead!
Most of the energy in any cell, cancer cell, heart cell, etcetera, it's the proton motive gradient across the membrane that determines whether or not that cell's gonna be alive. You need

183

any ATP for that. If the ATP dissipates, the cell will just die. Going through apoptosis or whatever.

You, as the cell, have to then determine „Where's my ATP coming from? How am I going to keep those pumps going?" And if fermentation becomes a replacement, therefore I'm going to need a lot of extra fermentable fuels to make up the loss of the energy that I'm not getting out of OxPhos.

So oncogenes have to turn on because they are the transcription factors that upregulate the transporters for glucose and glutamine. You're bringing in two alternative fuels to make up the difference, and therefore the genetic behavior of the cell begins to change.

Because the cell is now using damaged respiration, you throw out a lot of reactive oxygen species (ROS), from the damaged respiratory system - and they're mutagenic and carcinogenic! So the nuclear genome gradually collects all these different mutations and defects, coming from the ROS of the mitochondria!

But at the same time, the cell is not dying from this ROS because it's being protected by the fermentation pathways of glucose and glutamine.

Dr. Attia:
How much of that lactate is leaving the cell and going back to the liver, to undergo the Cori cycle?

Prof. Seyfried:
A lot of it does.

Dr. Attia:
Has anyone ever looked at patients who have a very, very high tumor burden and seeing if they appreciably have higher serum lactate levels?

Prof. Seyfried:
Yes, blood cancers have been examined.

In fact, there have been some patients who have had various leukemias, where they died of lactic acidosis, from so much lactic acid being produced by the tumor cells. A couple of papers reported on that, lactic acidosis from massive leukemias. Okay?

So, the leukemia: The same thing, it's a blood cell. Their mitochondria are defective, so they're throwing out a lot of lactic acid.

Dr. Attia:

That's a confusing one because I could come up with another explanation:

In very severe leukemias you could also create multiple end organ ischemia, just due to the defective nature of the... The white blood cells could actually cause capillary damage. That lactic acidosis could actually be from other organs.

Prof. Seyfried:
That's true, and the paper that I read seemed to focus on the lactic acidosis from the cancer cells themselves. But it doesn't rule out what you just said.

Dr. Attia:
Yeah, and we I don't know how you'd quantify the distinction.

Prof. Seyfried:
You're right, with a solid tumor, seeing a lot of lactic acid in the bloodstream... The Cori cycle clears it out pretty quick. So you're gonna be taking that lactic acid and making glucose again from it.

Dr. Attia:
Do tumor cells upregulate the machinery? I believe MC t2 is the lactate transporter. Do they upregulate that specifically?

Prof. Seyfried:
Yeah, it's upregulated, and so is lactic acid. LDH A, lactic acid dehydrogenase A. Which converts pyruvate to lactic acid. Rather than B.

So most cancer cells do not have elevated levels. This is why some people say

„Oh, cancer cells can burn lactic acid!“

„Where? They burning it?“

„Well, because the cancer cells are taking it back in“

No, that's bullsh*t. If it can't put pyruvate into the mitochondria, it's pumping out lactic acid. How is it possible...

[...1:35:40-1:35:55 very fast and unfortunately unintelligable biochemical details, see and listen to the video for clarification in the sources section]

Dr. Attia:
...because otherwise the hydrogen ion would poison the cell.

Prof. Seyfried:
Yeah, the whole thing is upregulated. Mono carboxylic acid transporters. And they also take in ketones. Don't forget that same transporter brings in ketones!

So when you go into ketogenic diets, the MCts are upregulated as well, you're bringing in more ketone bodies now.

Dr. Attia:

There's an irony for you, right there. The thing that you use to bring in ketones is giving you the exit for lactate, which protects the cell from the harm of the acidosis that comes with the hydrogen ion...

Prof. Seyfried:

...in the micro environment of the tumor, it's a real mess!

So some of the lactic acid is persisting, the hydrogen ions are persisting... until they can ooze out into the local bloodstream and get back to the liver that way. But otherwise, it's going to be a real acidic mess, which then contributes further to the fermentation behavior of the cells.

They're fermenting, right? So they don't need blood vessels! This is why the anti-angiogenic field has failed.

They said „We will target the blood vessels - and therefore the cancer cells will die because they can't get the oxygen". But the cancer cell doesn't need that! It doesn't need the blood vessels, it can ferment.

Dr. Attia:

Did you know Judah Folkman? You guys were basically neighbors.

Prof. Seyfried:

Yeah, I knew him. He came down here, he gave a talk. He targeted some unusual kinds of cancers with his anti-angiogenic strategy. But Napoleone Ferrara, I believe, was the guy who started taking that all off.

He even came to a meeting, he said „None of this stuff is working." This is why Avastin doesn't work. As I wrote „Avoid it like the plague!" It's a stupid drug, it was taken off the market for breast cancer because it was harming more people than it was helping.

But: They still use it for brain cancer!

Dr. Attia:

Do they still use it for colon answer as well?

Prof. Seyfried:

I don't know of colon cancer, but certainly for brain cancer. What are you guys doing? You're targeting the blood vessels and then forcing these cells to spread throughout your whole brain.

Dr. Attia:
For the reader's information: Avastin is an anti-angiogenic drug, this was a Genentech blockbuster.

Prof. Seyfried:
Yeah, Bevacizumab is the name of the drug, and they still use it! I think it' s despicable to consider anybody using that. I mean, if they knew the biology of the problem, they would never do that.

It's already been a bust in all the brain cancer studies that I've seen. In fact, my friends have told me that, who work on this.

Dr. Attia:
It's generally been priced out of use, certainly outside of the US. I don't think any third party payors would cover it. And it's a very expensive drug, it's about $100,000 a year drug!

Prof. Seyfried:
Yes, and all it does is contribute to the invasive behavior of these tumor cells.

Dr. Attia:
You're basically driving this idea, which I haven't wrapped my head around yet, that is:
You're actually enhancing the promotion of the hypoxic factors that are giving cancer some of its selective benefit?

Prof. Seyfried:
Yeah! And don't forget the cells that are invading which are coming from disrupted microglia in the brain. Macrophages, they will invade. They already have the capacity to do this. They live without blood vessels.

So you're facilitating the invasive behavior! This has been seen on histological preparations, brains that have been looked at after Avastin. They found tumor cells spread through everywhere in the brain - rather than clustered in one area. It's like they've just gone everywhere!

But when you look at the radiographic images, it looks good because you don't see that. The necrotic area that you would normally see. The image looks a little bit better.

You tell the patient „Looks like it's working" - but the overall survival is no different. Sometimes it's even less!

It's a false image of what's going on. You can't see the big central area, it's very vague and diffuse. „Yeah, it looks like this thing is working" – that just gives the guy false hope. Look at the overall survival statistics, they're abysmal.

Dr. Attia:

I want to go back to something you said a moment ago. You said macrophage, which reminded me of a point you brought up earlier:

The idea that the macrophage themself may be responsible for actual metastatic behavior. Can you say a bit more about that?

Prof. Seyfried:

Well, this is a concept that goes all the way back to a researcher from 1906 in Germany, in colon or melanoma, I can't remember the tissue.

He was actually observing fusion behavior between the neoplastic cells and the cells of our immune system. Then claimed that he thinks after fusion event, that these cells become much more aggressive and much more dispersive than before.

This was then solidified by the work of John Pollock at Yale University, where he did some beautiful experiments. Showing that malignant melanoma is actually a macrophage disease, they are the result of fusion hybridization.

This was then further established by Melissa Wong, her group at the Portland Medical Center, beautiful work. Showing in the colon, how macrophages were fusing with neoplastic stem cells, forming these hybrid cells.

And we know that all these metastatic cancers are highly fermentative. We know that, that's a fact. They're all highly fermentative - and they're all very, very invasive.

They spread, they migrate through the blood-brain barrier, they migrate everywhere. They just invade... these are all behaviors of macrophages.

Dr. Attia:

When you say fusion... so you have a neoplastic cell that is above the basement membrane, and you have a macrophage.

Tell me what the fusion actually is: Are they fusing genetic material? Or are they just fusing cytoplasmic material, what's actually happening?

Prof. Seyfried:

Well, it's combination of both, actually. So cells of our immune system are extremely fusogenic. They do wound healing. Like, you'll see multinucleated giant cells in a lot of parts of our bodies during wound healing.

188

In cancer cells, you also find a lot of these multinucleated kinds of cells.

Our body recognizes wounding as an acute problem, and the immune system will come into that local area to facilitate wound healing. And when the wound persists, sometimes these cells will fuse with each other, and fuse with other cells in the micro environment to facilitate wound healing.

The problem is: If you have an epithelial cell, like a breast cell or a colon cell, that is becoming neoplastic, becoming dysmorphic in its growth regulatory, and it's fermenting...

But it doesn't have the capacity to grow anywhere outside of that local area.

So our immune cells come into this lesion, if you will, that's persisting. The immune cell throws out growth factors and cytokines to facilitate wound healing.

The problem is those factors are also facilitating the growth of the neoplastic cell. So the neoplastic cell is dysregulated, but the very cell that's coming in to try to correct the wound is now provoking the cell to grow even more.

Dr. Attia:

But what is the wound that the macrophage is coming in for? Because the neoplastic cell has not yet violated the membrane beneath it.

Prof. Seyfried:

No, but it throws out lactic acid and creates a kind of a hypoxic micro area. Because lactic acid is a signal of hypoxia. It's a signal of some sort of damage! And you're not supposed to have pockets of build-up lactic acid in parts of your body.

Normally, if this does happen, if we have a contusion or a cut, cells of our monocytes mass migrate out of the bloodstream. They go into the wound, clear up the debris, kill the bacteria - and then move out of that section, go back to local lymph nodes and sit there, in the event that you need it again.

So these cells are part and parcel of the correction of the wound. The problem is: If you have a colon lesion or a breast lesion from an occluded milk duct or whatever, you have population of cells that will start to proliferate. Creating a damage to the local micro environmen, signaling to our immune system there's something going on here!

Dr. Attia:

Right, so when the monocyte gets out and differentiates, the macrophage goes to this now poorly differentiated cell... why doesn't it just kill that cell, nonspecifically? Because this is just a macrophage.

Prof. Seyfried:
Well, macrophages aren't designed to kill cells. They're designed to kill bacteria that may be in the micro environment. Don't forget, they're a wound healing cell.

Dr. Attia:
But going back to the bruise example: You get a contusion in your thigh, the macrophage does play a role in clearing that cellular debris.

Prof. Seyfried:
Yes.

Dr. Attia:
So why doesn't it just effectively do same thing with the cancers? Or with the soon-to-be cancer?

Prof. Seyfried:
Because the cell is not recognized as such. It looks like it's a part of the local normal epithelial cells. It's not looking as if this is a foreign invader, it looks like a regular epithelial cell that's proliferating.

Don't forget, we replace ourselves by proliferation.

Dr. Attia:
But the lactate secretion, what got it there in the first place - wouldn't that tell the macrophage hey, something's still wrong here?

Prof. Seyfried:
This cell is hardwired to do what it's supposed to do. It's not thinking „Oh, let me problem-solve this issue!" It's not a problem-solving cell, it's hardwired to respond to a particular environmental issue.

Dr. Attia:
I see. So you're saying, the lactate is the fire alarm that got it there. But then when it gets there, it doesn't see the fire?

Prof. Seyfried:
Well, it tries to put out the fire. But the problem is the molecules that are used to put out the fire are actually stimulating the growth of the cell that shouldn't be growing. So it's out of context.

Dr. Attia:
Okay. So how does this facilitate metastasis, rather than just local advancement?
Prof. Seyfried:
Right. At what point in this protracted process, does this now spring to become a metastatic lesion? Over a controlled proliferative abnormality, that's not yet breaking through the basement membrane? We don't know.

Sometimes this can happen very fast. Sometimes it takes a long period of time. Because we have these certain cancer cells, called cancer of unknown primary. They're highly metastatic but nobody knows where the hell they came from. They're very highly invasive.

Then, we have other cells that will... Well, he had a lesion there a long time, for several years. This thing never healed – and eventually explodes into a metastatic lesion. We don't know at what point... it varies from one person to the next.

We know their biology, they're fusogenic cells. There's massive amounts of biology to show that macrophages are very fusogenic cells. They can fuse with themselves or with other fibroblasts. They can fuse with a variety of different cells. Usually, that's part of the healing process, to facilitate wound healing.

But if you fuse with a stem cell that has already a defective respiratory systems, you would then dilute the cytoplasm of the cell that you fused it with - and it fuses again and again!

You eventually dilute the normal mitochondria in the macrophage and you replace it with the abnormal mitochondria from the cells that you're fusing with. Then leading to a cell with dysregulated growth properties.

How many mutations would it take to do that?

We don't know because there's some metastatic cells that don't have any mutations... if you can believe it. Using deep sequencing, they haven't found any mutations in some of these cells!

But they're fermenting and they're spreading. They have their growth dysregulated.
Dr. Attia:
Wait! How is their growth dysregulated without a mutation?
Prof. Seyfried:

You have cells that are carcinogenic, that are tumorigenic, that have no mutations. Baker pointed this out. It's like people can't believe this.

On the other hand, we have skin cells loaded with so-called driver mutations that never form a tumor.

So this linkage between the number of mutations and the type of cancer, there's so many flaws in this.

There are cancer cells that have been looked at, that are highly invasive and metastatic - and they can't find the mutations in there! That's not common, but it happens.

It's a violation to the whole concept.

In glioblastoma: There are some tumors that have been found, that have none of the driver mutations. None of them, none of the abnormalities that you would have expected, that are found in others.

So there's a break linkage between mutated... You don't need new mutations to cause a metastatic lesion. That doesn't mean that a metastatic lesion has no mutations.

Dr. Attia:
Maybe I'm asking a different question.

Okay, say two women have breast cancer. And, for all intents and purposes, they have very similar patterns of mutations in their breast cancer. Let's just make it easy and say that their hormonally similar. They're ER-PR positive, HER2-negative breast cancers.

Both women present as stage T to N1. So they've got a 5 centimeter tumor, and they've got two lymph nodes or one lymph node. They both have a resection.

Ten years later, one of them is still disease-free, the other one has died from brain metastasis. Which were presumably seeded before the primary tumor was resected 10 years earlier. It's not a sloppy surgery where they didn't get part of the cancer.

What I'm hearing you say is: Yes, one of them could undergo metastasis, while the other one did not - even though their primary tumors looked very similar. Is that correct?

Prof. Seyfried:
Yes, that's correct.

What we find now with a number of papers is that the needle biopsies that you use to diagnose the tumors can create a even more aggressive wounded situation in the micro environment of the tumor. Leading to the phenomenon of inflammatory oncotaxis, which facilitates the fusion.

In other words: By looking at the tumor with a needle biopsy to make the diagnosis, you put that patient potentially at risk for causing a metastatic lesion. And then, when you look at the profile, you say „Well, this doesn't look too bad..."

Dr. Attia:
But wait, wait. Let's say we do that - we're gonna immediately resect that tumor anyway. How quickly does this process take place?

Because the wound is between the outside world and the tumor, not between the tumor and the inside world, necessarily. Especially if that tumor is going to come out within a few weeks, right?

Prof. Seyfried:
Yeah. Still, we know from a number of studies that needle biopsies can facilitate - in some patients - the invasion of cells into the local environment and spread. We know this. This has been reported in the literature for breast, for colon, for liver, for brain.

The very act of stabbing this growth can...

Dr. Attia:
Maybe I misunderstood: You're saying that a woman who has a needle biopsy of her breast who then goes on to get a lumpectomy, has that increased her risk of brain metastasis?

Prof. Seyfried:
Well, it wouldn't be brain metastases right away. That brain metastases, the secondary metastatic behavior, has taken a while. It's not just the brain.

Dr. Attia:
How does needle a biopsy increase the risk of that?

Prof. Seyfried:
A needle biopsy creates a more inflamed condition. That's why it's called inflammatory oncotaxis. This was one of the reasons why they got rid of the morcellation procedure, because this is what was happening:

These women were dying from metastatic cancer from morcellation. It's kind of a machine that used to be made by *Johnson & Johnson* for removing uterine polyps. Well, you've taken a polyp and you're grinding it up, creating inflammatory oncotaxis.

There might have been one polyp out of a thousand that would have this...

Dr. Attia:

Right, but that's very different...

I'm asking a very specific question, because here's my fear: What I don't want is anybody who's got a breast lesion, thinks now they can't have it biopsied. I think that's a very different case than the example.

Prof. Seyfried:

Well, the evidence is clear. That it can happen in some cases, not all cases. Not everybody who goes under a needle biopsy is gonna have metastatic cancer.

Dr. Attia:

That's not the question. I mean, what I'm asking is: If you take a thousand women... it's a thought experiment:

You take a million women with an identical breast cancer. You take half a million of them, and you just do the resection. And the other half a million, you do a needle biopsy to confirm the diagnosis, then you do a resection.

Are you saying in the half a million women that had a resection following a biopsy, their probability of metastatic cancer later on is greater?

Prof. Seyfried:

I think so. But I can't be sure because that exact experiment hasn't been done, okay? I'm basing it on what is already known about needle biopsies facilitating the spread of the tumor.

Dr. Attia:

Again, I'm just being critical of this because feel very strongly about not causing panic in people. But I think those data are about needle tract seeding.

For example like as you said, you have a liver biopsy, you can get cancer cells through the tract even after... but that's very different from saying... because that that can be dealt with. But this very different.

Prof. Seyfried:

Well, I think this is from the perspective that I'm looking at. Now, I look at the brain, predominantly. It is not uncommon that when we remove a low-grade tumor, that within a shorter period

194

of time, it turns into a glioblastoma. This is the same phenomenon!

You're just doing it in a little bit larger scale, rather than just through a needle biopsy.

So you go in and you take out a low-grade tumor and all of a sudden, within a year or something, you've got glioblastoma! Sometimes even less.

And you say „What the hell happened here?"

Dr. Attia:

What's the control for that observation?

Meaning like another explanation would be: The person who has the stage 1 astrocytoma is more at risk for the stage 2, 3 or 4 astrocytoma.

Prof. Seyfried:

...from the operation itself. From the provocation of the micro environment.

Dr. Attia:

We'd have to have a group of those patients who don't undergo surgery.

Prof. Seyfried:

That's right. But who's doing that? Nobody's doing these experiments! Here's the situation:

What our philosophy is that if we shrink the tumor, whether it's a breast tumor - colon tumor or whatever - if we take away the fermentable fuels and shrink that tumor down, then it becomes a candidate for complete debulking.

Not diagnosing. Okay? We don't diagnose it by doing a biopsy. When you take a needle biopsy of a breast and you look at that...

Why are they doing that? They're doing it amazingly for two reasons.

- To try to diagnose what level of cancer you have. And then
- To give you a gene read out

As if this genes are gonna play some role. And whether or not you're gonna get a treatment.

Dr. Attia:

Yeah, for example in the case of doing a biopsy before a breast resection, there's value in knowing if a woman might benefit from neoadjuvant therapy for example, based on the receptor profile.

In other words, it might not just be the genes, right? Knowing that she's ER triple positive or negative might change what you do.

Prof. Seyfried:
Right, right. I guess it could. But the bottom line is:

Why don't you assume that you have a problem? Why don't you just put that patient on metabolic therapy and shrink that tumor down? And then, do a non-invasive check. With imaging only.

Did the border's change, from the metabolic intervention? And then just debulk it completely.

The probability of cure is going to be better, in my mind, than if you do a needle biopsy without doing the debulking, just to say Let's look at this.

How long after the needle biopsy do you put that patient at risk for possibly seeding a cell that gets to a lymph node, that then can spread out - and later you get brain metastases, liver metastases or whatever else can happen from these cancers.

So the question is: Why put anybody at risk? If we know, we have evidence from the literature, to say that is a possibility. Why would we want to put anyone at risk for that? Unless the information you get from the needle biopsy is going to be a curative procedure. And a lot of times it's not! It's just for diagnosis procedures.

Now today, we're using all these gene screens, $7,200 to tell somebody what kind of gene profile their cancer has - and that may no longer be relevant after you've taken a needle biopsy from the very tissue you're doing it from. Because people should do metabolic therapy, for which this gene stuff is completely useless.

Dr. Attia:
Yeah, I think that makes sense. I guess, I'm a bit confused by the idea.

Prof. Seyfried:
Yes, these are controversial issues. I'm looking at it from the point of the biological processes that are taking place from these procedures. And knowing that I've seen literature on lung cancer, I've seen liver cancer, certainly for brain.

Dr. Attia:
I mean, there are so many potential arguments.

You look at one of the most metastatic cancers of all time, is pancreatic cancer. Right? It's almost uniformly fatal! And yet, up until recently, very infrequently biopsied. It's a very difficult biopsy, you have do it with an ERCP.

Prof. Seyfried:
That's true.

Dr. Attia:
You can still have incredibly aggressive metabolic cancers which are not biopsied often. And then conversely, you look at a GBM. A very aggressive cancer that John McCain just passed away from.

That's only locally metastatic. It never leaves the CNS, does it?

Prof. Seyfried:
Oh, yeah. It does.

Dr. Attia:
Where does it go?

Prof. Seyfried:
It goes to bone, it goes to liver. Nobody looks at the...

Dr. Attia:
What percentage of patients die from those?

Prof. Seyfried:
Not many. But when they look, they find the metastatic cells. This was one of the big things, this is how we discovered the macrophage origin of the cancer:

We started looking and saying „How many people do autopsies of organs on people who've died from glioblastoma?“

Dr. Attia:
And what did you find?

Prof. Seyfried:
There's a hundred articles in the literature with metastatic GBM to various organs, for people dying.

People say „Well, it doesn't happen that often“. You know why? They died from the GBM before they started recognizing they have metastatic liver cancer.

But when you look at livers and kidneys and these other organs from patients who have died from GBM - those studies that have looked have found cancer!

So clearly, these cells are coming out of the brain and they're getting into the other organs. The problem is the patients aren't

197

living long enough to have a problem. What are we worrying about the guy's liver, when his brain is starting to swell up from from all the treatments they're giving him?

I mean, in 12 months most people are dead. But there's over 100 articles in the scientific literature, showing extracranial metastasis of glioblastoma.

And people ignore it! They're ignoring it like they're ignoring that the mitochondria are damaged in cancer cells.

Dr. Attia:
Well, I guess that'd be a more forgivable thing to ignore. Because I'm not convinced it necessarily changes the story. The mitochondrial one is a much more interesting question. I mean, that to me...

Of all the things we've talked about today, that's the one that has me scratching my head the most. And I am wondering in 2018:

This should be something that's not debated. This would be like debating whether DNA is necessary to make RNA. Like, that discussion was settled in the 50s and anyone who disputes that today is sort of disputing the shape of the earth.

So I guess to me, given the stakes here, I would love to figure out why people aren't answering this question.

Prof. Seyfried:
Well, let's look at the situation from even a greater distance: In the United States, we have over 1,600 people a day dying from cancer, right? This is horrific! There's over a half a million people a year, 1,600 people a day dying from cancer.

Obviously, there's something seriously wrong! There's something massively wrong with what we're doing with this disease.

When we talk about needle biopsies... we're talking about this, we're talking about that. The issue is we have 1,600 people a day dying.

Why are all these people dying from cancer?

It's either we have a fundamental misunderstanding of what the nature of the disease is. Were mistreating it. We're treating it as something other than what it actually is.

The debate that you mentioned... The dead people are the consequences of the fundamental misunderstanding of the process of the biology of the disease.

What I'm arguing is: Now, understanding the biology of the disease, we have the potential to drop the death rate by more than 50% in 10 years! There's no question about it.

If you stop doing half of the stuff that we're doing to these cancer patients, looking at the biology and the nature of the disease, how to best go about this strategically... I think we can drop the death rate by 50%.

We're doing stupid things. Right? To needle biopsy tumor cells for gene profiling, that has no relevance to the nature of the disease. That's just one.

Prof. Seyfried:
Just to go back to that because, I'm sorry. I really want to make sure people aren't gonna refusing their biopsies. Have we seen an increase in the rate of metastases in the era of needle biopsy for genetic sequencing?

I mean, we could go back and look at the death rate from cancer 50 years ago before anybody was doing this, and it was the same. Probably.

Prof. Seyfried:
I don't want to say... I just want to say that every year, we have more and more dead people. And the increase is faster than the general population increase, okay?

So we had a 3.8% increase in death rates.

Dr. Attia:
Is that actually true? Is the age adjusted, population adjusted mortality of cancer today higher than it was 50 years ago? I think it's about 3 or 4% lower.

Prof. Seyfried:
Well, I just did the last 5 years, from 2013 to 2017.

Dr. Attia:
But to test this hypothesis, we'd want to take an even longer time period.

Prof. Seyfried:
Well, every year it goes up. There's no year that we have fewer. The dead people are piling up. You know, when I look at the numbers and I say „Okay, what was the of population increase in the United States over the last 5 years? - and according to the demographics it's 2.9%.

Over the same period, how many cancer deaths did we have?

Dr. Attia:

Correct, but again... I don't know my epidemiology well enough to make this case, but I'm gonna try anyway:

Isn't the growth in population more a function of the input of people, meaning birth rate - rather than the people who are getting cancer, which are the older folks?

Prof. Seyfried:
Well, we have younger people, too.

Dr. Attia:
Right, but the majority...

Prof. Seyfried:
...are older folks, yes.

Dr. Attia:
So I'm not sure that that population argument would answer that question.

Prof. Seyfried:
I think all you have to look at is the numbers of people that are dying from the disease. I mean that 1,600 a day number, that's a fact.

Dr. Attia:
It's a fact and it's a tragic fact!

I guess a 50% reduction in the mortality of this disease in 10 years is a very bold statement, given that we've seen about a 3% reduction in cancer mortality in 50 years, Which, I think you're arguing, is unacceptable and understandable.

Prof. Seyfried:
Yeah, I'm looking at it from from the tragedy. In China, it's 8,100 people a day dying from cancer. I mean, that's the number over there, they have a bigger population. But the problem is it's now surpassed heart disease in their country as the number one cause of death.

Clearly, whatever we're doing it's not working.

And yes, 50%! If you did what we think you need to do to manage this disease, looking at it from the biology of the disease - I would not be shocked if we had a 50% reduction in 10 years.

Dr. Attia:
So normally, I ask people what their dream experiment would be. But I want to ask you 2 experiments. I want to ask you this question twice:

The first time I'll ask you this question will be the easier one, because it'll be the clinical trial. So what would be the dream clinical trial to test the hypothesis that says we can reduce the mortality of cancer by 50%?

What would you want to put head-to-head, to definitively answer that question?

Prof. Seyfried:
If we do metabolic therapy... at all. If we do it at all, it's standard of care versus standard of care plus metabolic therapy. That is what we are allowed to do right now, But:

We're missing the critical control group: Metabolic therapy without standard of care!

Dr. Attia:
So tell me what the experiment would be. Let's use breast cancer as an example.

Prof. Seyfried:
Okay, breast cancer. You have your standard whatever, what you're doing today. You know, a lot of people are dying of metastatic breast cancer.

So we're gonna take metabolic therapy and we're gonna combine it with standard of care. Which is what the group in Turkey is doing.

Dr. Attia:
How would you integrate that? Let's talk about how you would do it, not necessarily have it's being done now.

How would you - for the purpose of the experiment - integrate standard of care and metabolic therapy?

Prof. Seyfried:
We would have one group use the chemo, and then we would have people on metabolic therapy.

Dr. Attia:
You would do those in parallel?

Prof. Seyfried:
You would have some patients that would be treated only with the standard of care, which would be our control group.

And then we would have people treated with the standard of care plus reducing blood sugars, elevating ketones, and targeting the energy metabolism.

Dr. Attia:
Would that include things like metformin, TCA, other things like that?

Prof. Seyfried:

It could.
Dr. Attia:
Hyperbaric oxygen chamber treatments?
Prof. Seyfried:
Yes, definitely. That's what we're doing in Turkey. However, we're doing the lowest dose of chemo that we can use, to still be in compliance with the law.
Dr. Attia:
And now your metabolic therapy alone group?
Prof. Seyfried:
That group would be everything that's proposed in our press pulse concept: So we downregulate the glucose first. Shrink the tumor, make the microenvironment less inflamed, less angry.
Dr. Attia:
Specifically, tell me what would be done in that group. Would these patients be on ketogenic diet?
Prof. Seyfried:
First we'd lower their blood sugar gradually, depending on the status of the individual.

So you'd go into lowering their blood sugar and elevating their ketones by putting them to therapeutic ketosis essentially. Yes, a ketogenic diet.

A lot of these people also have multiple other metabolic abnormalities. They have type 2 diabetes, they've got triglyceridemia, they have all kinds of other things - besides having cancer. Bringing them into a state of therapeutic ketosis.
Dr. Attia:
How do you define that? Is that defined by the amount of glucose and ketones?
Prof. Seyfried:
By the glucose ketone index (GKI) that we published. We published a paper on this.
Dr. Attia:
What's the ratio of glucose to ketones in this index?
Prof. Seyfried:
Close to 1.0 or below. If we can get it. This is where the millimolar of ketones and the millimolar of glucose are about the same.
Dr. Attia:
People hit that somewhere between 3 and 4 millimolar, I'm guessing?

Prof. Seyfried:
It could be, it depends on the individual. Because some people have higher glucose, higher ketones - and yet, they still have the same ratio.

Dr. Attia:
The only time I've been able to be at a 1-1 ratio was when I'm not eating anything!

Prof. Seyfried:
Yeah. Well, it's variable from one person to the next. That's the other thing too, we have to be very careful about:

There's a lot of cancer patients for which it's very hard to get to that one ratio. You're a young healthy guy, guys that are young and healthy can get well below one. Women are better than men. We've done some studies on that.

But cancer patients are freaked out because they have anxiety, and anxiety elevates corticosteroids. You have a tougher time bringing the glucose down.

We also institute besides and within the press treatments, ketone supplementation - Dominic D'Agostino is talking about that – along with the ketogenic diet .

And then, we have stress management. Which includes music therapy, yoga therapy... There's a variety of ways to reduce emotional stress. That's a very important part of the management.

You have to let the patient know that their disease is not terminal, that their lowering of the stress is going to make the medicine and the treatments work better.

So once we get the patient into metabolic ketosis, now we have options. Now we can start using insulin therapy to bring the blood sugar's down lower.

We can put them into hyperbaric oxygen, which creates oxidative stress predominantly in the tumor cells and not in the normal cells. The normal cells are burning ketones. That reduces oxidative stress.

Dr. Attia:
When you say insulin therapies, do you mean actual insulin?

Prof. Seyfried:
Yeah. We're testing that now. The Germans used to do that years ago. But we don't think we have to put people into metabolic comas to do this. We think we can do it without it, we're testing

it now. I'm working on it now as we speak. We have these experiments going next door.

You don't want to use insulin therapy, unless you're in therapeutic ketosis. You don't want to go into a hyperbaric chamber, unless you're in therapeutic ketosis.

Then we would pulse with drugs that target glutamine. And together, you're removing the antioxidant capacity of the tumor, making it vulnerable to hyperbaric oxygen.

Dr. Attia:
How much can these drugs lower local levels of glutamine?

Prof. Seyfried:
Enough to slaughter the tumor cells!

Dr. Attia:
I don't know enough about this. Is that a 50% reduction that's necessary to do that? Because you're getting about a 50% reduction in glucose, based on the therapy you've described.

Prof. Seyfried:
We want to lower the glucose even further, you can do that. With targeting glutamine, it's got to be pulsed. Because you can't chronically reduce glutamine.

Dr. Attia:
Acutely, how much do you lower it?

Prof. Seyfried:
We can lower it quite effectively! Don't forget: The cancer cell is absolutely dependent on this fuel. The normal cells, they can burn the ketones also. So they're not gonna be energy deprived completely, whereas the tumor cell will be energy deprived completely.

Dr. Attia:
Are there some cancer cells that preferentially utilize ketones?

Prof. Seyfried:
No cancer cell can use ketones. You have to have a good mitochondria. A cancer cell that would have some oxidative capacity, a small amount of oxidative capacity, could burn some ketones. But most can't.

Most of the most aggressive cancer cells can't burn ketones because their mitochondria are defective.

That's why it's selective. It selects for enhancing the vitality of the normal cell, while putting the cancer cell at a competitive disadvantage. The ketones are not to kill cancer cells, they do provide the normal cells with a fuel as an alternative to glucose.

There are many experiments like this. If you take cancer cells and grow them in a dish without glucose and glutamine, just ketones, they die. The normal cells don't, the normal cells can survive on the ketones, without the glucose and glutamine.

We're selectively marginalizing these tumor cells because of their metabolic incapabilities. But it has to be done strategically, over time.

Dr. Attia:
And where does the hyperbaric oxygen fit in? Is that part of the pulse? And how much of it?

Prof. Seyfried:
Yeah, that's a pulse therapy. We want to try to replace radiation therapy with hyperbaric oxygen. Because the mechanisms of cell death will be very similar.

Dr. Attia:
So how many atmospheres and for how long?

Prof. Seyfried:
We do it at 2.5 atmospheres and we're doing it for 90 minutes every day, something like this. It's designed to kill the tumor cells by oxidative stress. The same way radiation therapy would work.

A lot of times radiation doesn't work because the cells are in a hypoxic environment. So why are they in such a hypoxic environment? Because they're fermenting, they're blowing out all these waste products. Got to clean that all up. That micro environment has to be brought back to a normal state.

Therapeutic ketosis: We published several papers showing that it's

- An powerful anti-inflammatory therapy,
- It makes the micro environment less inflamed,
- It's pro-apoptotic,
- It's anti-angiogenic.

So you're killing all these bad blood vessels and replace the with normal blood vessels, that the normal cells will be able to use. It's reconfiguring the micro environment, while putting stress and killing tumor cells.

Now the tumor becomes more and more vulnerable, and now it becomes more and more damaged by drugs that are going to chip away at the surviving cells.

It's not something we're gonna do like a bull in a china shop - it's going to be a gradual degrading of the tumor.

Dr. Attia:

And where does the surgery take place here? Is the surgery taking place before all of this happens?

Prof. Seyfried:

No, the surgery would take place at some midpoint. Okay? The midpoint would be where the surgeon now looks at the tumor and says „I can take care of this!"

It's not going to be a diffuse mass, it's not gonna be an angry inflamed thing - where you have to cut out half the guys' colon, in order to get what the surgeon thinks is the part of the cancer.

No, this thing will be now much more shriveled. We've seen it, it's much less angry. It's more demarcated, you can see it on the histological slides.

You can see... „What the hell happened to this tumor? How come it's smaller? How come the margins are more sharply defined?" Because you took away the inflammation that was being driven by the fermentation fuels.

So you're shrinking this tumor down, now the surgeon comes in and can potentially cure these people, that were maybe not curable in the past.

This is why I'm saying we can reduce the death rate by 50% - if you view the tumor as a metabolic problem rather than a genetic problem. The gene mutations are all downstream epiphenomena, they're red herrings.

Even Vogelstein... he still claims it's a genetic disease but he also says we're never going to cure the disease by targeting the genes, as there are too many mutations, all this kind of stuff.

But we can do that with metabolic therapy - we can actually eliminate the cancer! Based on metabolic therapy. It's a process.

Who's trained to do this? No one! I mean, we need physicians to be trained to do this.

They've been trained to give high doses of radiation, without killing the patient... poisoning these poor people with drugs that are very toxic. Trying to keep them alive so they don't die from the treatments.

This is absurd! Why are you using radiation and chemo in the first place?

„Well, we have to stop proliferation!" Well, if they can't generate energy, they're going to stop proliferating, as they're gonna die!

Dr. Attia:
What is the experiment, the clinical trial, that you're involved in in Turkey?

Prof. Seyfried:
Yeah, so what my colleagues in Turkey do is: They use chemo, but they use the lowest possible dose.

Dr. Attia:
Is it for breast cancer?

Prof. Seyfried:
All cancers. In fact, the results are the same. All cancers are the same disease. They're all fermenters. Once you know that they're all dependent on these two fuels, then all you have to do is target the two fuels to eliminate them.

The question is: How can you target the fuels without harming the rest of the body? And that's the press-pulse concept. So we know we can press things constantly, without harming the body.

But we have the glutamine issue. Because we don't want to deprive our normal immune system and gut system of the very fuel needed to provide normal physiology in those tissues. This is why we have to pulse the glutamine issue.

How many glutamine drugs are there? Well, there are some. But the one that works the best for us is DON.

Dr. Attia:
Are there any that are in clinical trials in the United States?

Prof. Seyfried:
Yeah, there's a couple. There's a few names of them. They target various aspects of the glutaminolysis pathway.

The problem is we have a drug... it's a dirty drug. It hits multiple pathways of glutamine metabolism and it seems to work better than all the other drugs. At least from our perspective, so far.

Dr. Attia:
Which drug is this?

Prof. Seyfried:

Again, it's the DON, the 6-diazo-5-oxo-L-nor-Leucine. It was used in clinical trials years ago, but it was partially effective only. But they weren't targeting... they weren't doing the full metabolic approach. If you don't do all the parts of the problem, the horse is going to get out. It's not going to be effective.

Today, no one anywhere on the planet is doing the kind of a therapy that we think we need to do, to make this all work. Now, there's bits and pieces of it...

Dr. Attia:
What are the drugs that are in current clinical trials that are targeting glutamine?

Prof. Seyfried:
Well there's BEPTS I believe, an acronym for another very complicated structure. And then, they're making DON-analogues that are supposedly less toxic.

What we found is: With the ketogenic diet, DON becomes far less toxic. You can use far lower doses.

I was talking to somebody the other day „Is it better to wait for a pharmaceutical company to build a new drug to target cancer? Or is it better to develop a way in which a previously very effective drug could be less toxic?"

So how many clinics in the country - in the world - are treating cancer as a metabolic disease? Using a strategy that will take away the two prime fermentable fuels for the disorder? The answer is no one! No one's doing this.

Dr. Attia:
This trial in Turkey is doing this?

Prof. Seyfried:
Well, they're not targeting the glutamine! They're doing these other processes. Protocols.

Dr. Attia:
So it's the glucose, the ketones, the hyperbaric oxygen - but not pulsing with glutamine?

Prof. Seyfried:
Yes, they are not doing the glutamine. Nobody's doing the glutamine.

We tried doing that in our Egyptian patient that we published recently. We used chloroquine and we used EGCG, which is a green tea extract. But they're not as powerful in the clinic.

Now, that poor guy, he just passed away... we were devastated by this. He lived 30 months - which is far longer than most people live with a glioblastoma.

He was doing really well on metabolic therapy. We pushed off the standard of care for 3 months. So we did surgery after 3 weeks of therapeutic ketosis, debulk the tumor. Most of it, because you never get all GBM.

Then we were forced into the radiation therapy after 3 months, even though the guy was doing remarkably well. We said „Why are we radiating?" „We have to because it's part of the standard of care." Even there, this was in Alexandria, Egypt.

And then, 6 or 8 months later, he starts developing a headache, his head starts to swell... and they did a decompression debulking.

They looked at the tissue, they weren't any tumor cells: He was dying from radiation necrosis that he took from the radiation!

This is why I'm very much against it. I think we're not going to make any major advance in brain cancer until we stop radiating people with the brain! Because you're creating a bigger problem, and this is leading to the demise of all these poor patients.

The survival after radiation is almost zero! In my mind, that's because they are doing radiation. In part. So whether they're dying from the tumor or radiation necrosis, they're going to be dying. They shouldn't be doing that in the first place!

The standards of care have to be dramatically changed in order to improve overall survival. So when I say we can drop death rates by 50% in 10 years, we're not only dropping death rates! We're massively increasing overall survival and quality of life at the same time.

I have a lot of anecdotal information with people who have been treated with metabolic therapy. They're living far longer, their quality of life is much better. And when they die, they die in a very peaceful way.

Some of my clinician friends have been telling me this: These guys that are on these metabolic therapies, their quality of life is really good up until about 2 weeks before they die.

Whereas the people doing standard of care never live as long and their quality of life is horrific!

Dr. Attia:

Do you think that metabolic therapies offer the potential for cure? Or just another therapeutic option?

Because if you want to reduce the death rate by 50%, it there's no leetime bias / therapeutic extension that's gonna do that. That is a paradigm shift in cure, not treatment!

Prof. Seyfried:

I think it's both. I think you're going to be able to extend overall survival dramatically. You're going to improve dramatically quality of life. And how do we know if we're cured?

The issue is that, if you die from a heart disease at 85 and you had cancer when you were 50, a so called a terminal disease...

Dr. Attia:

I think we could pick something simpler than that, right? If you are 10 years disease-free... to a first order approximation, you're cancer-free. If you had colon cancer 10 years ago, and 10 years later you die of a heart attack, I think it's safe to say you died of heart disease. Even if on autopsy, they find dormant cancer cells.

Prof. Seyfried:

Well, here's the situation: If you take standard of care and you live 10 years after you have ben „cured", then drop dead of a heart attack - was that heart attack the result of the cancer? Or of the treatment? If you look at it like that, you still died of cancer, more or less.

Because you also have to put into perspective what effect does the treatments have on your overall long-term survival as well.

So Dana-Farber down here, they just opened up a branch of medicine called Cancer Survivor Medicine. It appears that many people treated with standards of care are suffering horrificly from all these other diseases they never had - but for the fact that they were treated with all this toxic stuff.

So we would eliminate that.

Dr. Attia:

But I'm still, like... What's the proof of concept that the metabolic therapy can lead to a cure? Your hypothesis is that this gentleman in Alexandria, if he hadn't undergone radiation for the GBM, your belief is that he could have actually had a cure?

Prof. Seyfried:

I don't know. Because we can't know. Like you said, we'd have to wait 10 years to know that. So if we were to institute an aggressive metabolic program for managing cancer...

Dr. Attia:
But it seems GBM would be the place to do it, right? Because unfortunately, it is such a uniformly fatal cancer.

Prof. Seyfried:
It would be! It's fatal because of the treatment that they're giving, this combination of what they're doing to the patient, as well as the tumor.

Dr. Attia:
The problem clinically is that the mass effect doesn't give you a lot of flexibility to delay surgery. So between corticosteroids and radiation, when a patient...

When most patients present with GBM not as incidental findings, they have symptoms from the mass effect. So we have to be sympathetic to the clinicians in the conventional pathway, who are saying

„Look, I got Bob here. He's complaining, he's got hemiparalysis and he's got a GBM...!

The idea that we're gonna wait a month to put him on a ketogenic diet, when I need to either cut that thing out now, radiate him or or put him on corticosteroids.“

In other words, it's gonna be a very difficult thing to study.

Prof. Seyfried:
Well, it's a judgment call on the part of the neurosurgeon. So he looks at the data, do we have a watchful waiting period. I have spoken to many neurosurgeons, some of my friends are surgeons.

I said „What do we do here?“ He said „Occasionally, if you have a brain herniation possibility, the patient would be dead in a week if we don't do the debulking!“ That patient has to be debulked.

All right. But you don't have to give them steroids. You can just do debulking. Steroids will shrink the edema...

Dr. Attia:
Okay. Of the three, what would be the most evil in your mind, meaning metabolically evil? The radiation, the corticosteroids or the surgery?

Prof. Seyfried:
Oh clearly, the steroids and the radiation.

Dr. Attia:

So you're saying every GBM patient should go and have the resection - and then undergo metabolic therapy? Even though they're not technically going to be free of disease.

Prof. Seyfried:
Yeah, I think this is a strategy. The watchful waiting period will give the neurosurgeon an opportunity to do a greater debulking.

And there's a hundred articles in the literature showing that you'll live longer the more you can debulk the tumur.

So if we can shrink the tumor down like we did in our Egyptian patient: We waited 3 weeks! We put him under incredible therapeutic fasting, water only, a 900 calories ketogenic diet.

Dr. Attia:
900 calories? But not water only, right?

Prof. Seyfried:
Water only for the first 3 days, to get him into ketosis as fast as possible.

Then, he did an awake craniotomy, it was done very well. Then we pushed off the radiation therapy for 3 months. We didn't want to do that because the tumor was looking really good.

He had a correction of the midline shift, he was in good shape. So I think he suffered from the radiation. I think he didn't survive because of the radiation treatment.

Dr. Attia:
Do you think that GBM would be the best histology to study this in?

Prof. Seyfried:
Oh yeah. Because as you said, the survival is the hard endpoint.

Dr. Attia:
You're gonna see a signal if one's there.

Prof. Seyfried:
Yes. Then I've spoken to a lot of my friends, who think „Okay we have to debulk immediately, then we're going to go on metabolic therapy. We can push it off for two weeks and then do metabolic therapy." [Beforehand, if possible]

The thing we have to do is: We have to eliminate radiation! I think radiation is the biggest part of the problem. I think if you're doing metabolic therapy, you should eliminate radiation right away. I have no doubt about this.

This is one of the reasons why there's so few people surviving. It's because you are radiating. If you didn't radiate, you could survive a lot longer. I think with a metabolic therapy you can double, triple the amount of survival in GBM patients.

How do we know this? Because those patients that I know who rejected radiation and chemo, took surgery after two years or a year, they are doing well. They're out 4 years!

Dr. Attia:
There are GBM patients alive at 4 years?

Prof. Seyfried:
Yes, Pablo Kelly!

Dr. Attia:
Is this published?

Prof. Seyfried:
No, it's not published. But the guy has all the documentation. It's just that it's not yet published. (...)

In fact, he's gonna be giving a lecture after my lecture. He's a young guy, 25 years old. He says „I don't want radiation. I don't want chemo, I don't want any of that stuff. I don't want surgery!" Oh, you're gonna be dead in 3 to 6 months. This is what they told him! It's all in the news, it was in the newspapers.

I gave him the stuff on the metabolic therapy. I didn't know he was gonna live that long. I thought he was just gonna live a few extra months!

He comes back a long time later and he says I'm still alive! And there's a big newspaper article in the British newspapers about this guy who rejects all the medical stuff!

After two years he decides... he had an inoperable glioblastoma that now became operable, after metabolic therapy. So they debulked it. And now after another year, he doesn't have any tumor left!

He never had radiation, he never had chemo. He had surgery, very delayed. And they did a histological analysis after the debulking, which said yes, you did have a GBM. Because what a lot of people say „If you live that long, you didn't have GBM" – that's bullsh*t!

I mean, you're creating a situation that leads to the demise of those very people that you are trying to help. When you irradiate the brain, you free up massive amounts of glutamine by breaking the glutamine-glutamate cycle. So those tumor cells are sucking down massive amounts of glutamine.

Then you give the steroids to reduce the edema, which then elevates the blood sugar.

Dr. Attia:

I was going to give you two experiments, two dream experiments. So the second one would be... going back to sort of the more fundamental premise of this. Which is:

If resources were no constraint, how could one unambiguously make the case / test the hypothesis, that despite structural abnormalities in the mitochondria, the production of lactate (and the fermentation) is not purely for respiratory compensation?

In other words - we talked about this idea that says: You can have a structural deficit but it would still be functionally good enough.

How could that hypothesis be tested? Because that seems to be one of the central arguments here.

Prof. Seyfried:

Well, there are several ways we can look at this. If a cell can live with ketones, without glucose and glutamine, you'd obviously have some mitochondrial function that would keep them alive. Because they wouldn't be able to ferment.

Dr. Attia:

But let's, like... we're in a resource unconstraint world. So what are the dream experiments that would test that in humans...?

Prof. Seyfried:

Right, because a lot of these mechanisms would be tested in vitro. You can't do those kinds of experiments.

But the metabolic therapy that we have designed, Dom D'Agostino, myself, Joel Maroon who's the team surgeon for the Pittsburgh Steelers, neurosurgeon... George Yeo is a who's a prostate cancer oncologist. We all sat down and we built this press-pulse therapy.

If you deprive the tumor cells of their fermentable fuels and you essentially eliminate, you can't detect any more cancer in your body, that's based on the biology of what the problem is.

The dream experiments are to ferret that out mechanistically, in vitro. To prove that this is the case and we're doing that right now. When we target these things, these cells die. So you can put them in an environment where normal cells wouldn't die, so clearly what's going on here is that the mitochondria don't work properly.

I mean, it was shown in many papers. In fact, back in the 30s and 40s, they published beautiful papers, showing that the respiratory system of tumor cells is massively compromised. Okay, if that's the case, then they're surviving on fermentation. There's no other known biological system in the world that can provide alternative ATP.

Dr. Attia:
But yet, most people don't agree with that statement. So that's what I'm asking is:

What experiment could take the debate out of that very important question?

Prof. Seyfried:
Okay, they don't believe it. If I look at the data and you look at the data and we both come to the same conclusion - and this other guy looks at the same data and he says „I don't believe it!"...

Dr. Attia:
...then it tells me the data are not convincing enough, if everybody's acting in good faith.

Prof. Seyfried:
Well, then you have to ask about what's good faith?

Dr. Attia:
Or: What and where is the better data?

Prof. Seyfried:
Okay, here's the way I look at it: If science is a human activity, there are people who say things that are not true and everybody believes it. Right? But the issue here of course is that, it's one thing to say „Okay..."

We had a review on a paper, saying we know there's a massive biology on the role of cardiolipin on controlling the electron transport chain! There's dozens and dozens of papers on this.

The molecular biologists say „I don't believe it" – well, what don't you believe? What part of this massive amount of scientific evidence is it that you don't believe?!

„I'm unfamiliar with cardiolipin, therefore it can't be right." Well, that's not a reason to discount the evidence.

Dr. Attia:
Right, right.

Prof. Seyfried:

And when they write new papers up, why would you not cite Pete Peterson's massive compendium of evidence, saying mitochondria are abnormal - and you say mitochondria are normal? How does that jive with the massive amounts of evidence that say that it is not?

What I tried to do, in all my writings: I never tried to ignore an alternative fact to what I'm saying. I say „There is a fact that I'm not yet completely clear about - but I'm not going to ignore it."

You'll find in the scientific literature today, in the top journals, that they're ignoring massive evidence that doesn't support their position. And that's one of the problems.

Like we were saying, that this problem in cancer... all these top journals Cell, Science, Nature, up to 50% of the articles' findings can't be reproduced in other people's labs. This is a crisis in the field! What's going on here?

You're ignoring massive evidence that doesn't fit your particular mindset, so you'll just discount it.

I don't think it's any different than the geocentric / heliocentric model of the solar system. The Catholic Church refused to believe that the earth was not the center of the solar system, despite all the evidence that said it was. They just refused to believe it.

We have the exact same thing in the cancer field. You have massive evidence, showing that the mitochondria are structurally and functionally dysfunctional.

I don't want to believe it!

What can you do about that? What can you do about that, when you have the evidence to show that and the field chooses to ignore it? Is that any different than the geocentric / heliocentric system that we had? The difference today is that we have 1,600 people dying of this tragedy a day.

Dr. Attia:
I think the Catholic Church was basically relying on a religious framework, that was their counter argument. Their belief system was formed by something different. I think in the scientific field...

Prof. Seyfried:
Yeah. But when Galileo said „Please, look through the telescope" to document that Copernicus was right, they didn't want to look

216

in the telescope. They didn't want to look in the telescope, because it would disrupt their worldview.
Dr. Attia:
I think that's a fair statement. I guess, again, I would like to come back to this through the lens of...

I'd just love to know what the experiments are that could solve this. Because I view it as a stalemate.

If you're looking at a body of literature, they're looking at a different body of literature, and every time everybody looks at everybody else's body of literature, they say „Well, there's an alternative explanation for your hypothesis" – then, we're making no progress.

The answer to me is: You guys should collaborate and generate new experiments.
Prof. Seyfried:
That's why I think, knowing the biology of the disease as well as I think I do.... and we never can know completely everything because every human being is a different entity.

If we can increase overall survival and improve quality of life, massively advanced to what we're doing today, because we use a strategy based on what we understand to be the biological problem, and the results support that – then, I think, that right there is the advance!

And glioblastoma would be a wonderful case.
Dr. Attia:
So speaking of that: Realistically, when do you think that case report of these 4 year survivors will be published?
Prof. Seyfried:
I'm going to try when I talk to Pablo Kelly over there. I'd like to speak to the very physicians that actually took the data from him.
Dr. Attia:
Was it only one? I thought there were multiple patients.
Prof. Seyfried:
Well, there is Andrew Scarborough, who had a first couple of radiation sessions, then he said "No more of this!" He took no radiation, no chemo. He's still going. He had a stage 3 astrocytoma which is also quite lethal.

Then there's Alison Ganic, she's on the news. She has a website saying, that she survived GBM without this.

I have other anecdotal reports, based on what people have told me:

One poor guy, he had no money. No insurance. So they didn't treat or operate him because they wouldn't be able to get any revenue from this guy.

He just did the ketogenic diet, way back before even I was talking about it - and he's still alive! For 16 years!

Dr. Attia:

Did they eventually do surgery on him?

Prof. Seyfried:

They did surgery, but they didn't do anything else.

Again, these are anecdotal. But with Pablo, we have clear dats. So it's not like we don't have data from him. With a lot of these things, physicians would say „You can't do this. You can't do what what I'm asking you to do because it breaks the it violates the standard of care!" Okay?

The standard of care should never have been written in granite.

It should be flexible.

If you have something else that comes along that might be better, you think there would be an enthusiasm. No, we have not seen that. We tried to get this through the University of Pittsburgh, to try to do this. Through the advisory board, the IRB.

The IRB refused. They only might consider metabolic therapy after standard of care failed. But standard of care fails all the time!

„Why don't you try metabolic therapy as an alternative to standard of care?"

„No, we can't do that!"

„Why?"

„Well, because we can't do that."

„Why?!"

„Because we can't do that."

That means there's inflexibility. So we're up against firewalls after firewalls after firewalls, to try to change the way we continue.

They are doing all this gene screening, amounting to nothing. Because cancer is not a genetic disease!

218

So we have all these firewalls that are preventing us from moving forward the way we need to be moving forward. For a GBM patient, what do they have to lose?

There was a paper that just came out the other day, out of British Columbia Canada, carefully looking a survival for GBM.

They said it's woefully similar to the 1926 Bailey and Cushing paper! For Chrissake, I mean, what's going on here? You mean, in almost 100 years... John McCain passing away from GBM today, that's no different than if he had the tumor in 1926?!

That tells us we have a serious, serious problem - and I'm offering an alternative that might be able to change that. What is wrong with that? Why would I personally be attacked for something like this? So you tell me, I have to know what's going on here.

So I go up and I say „You can't irradiate the brain" - „Oh, you got to do it!"

Dr. Attia:

(...)

You've got to find advocates on the other side of this ledger. Meaning in terms of the thinking about this disease.

(...)

Prof. Seyfried:

I know, I'm speaking to people who want to set up these special clinics, special kind of treatment clinics where we can bring everything under the same roof. So you don't have to run, over to this place or that place. We take the patients that want to do metabolic therapy.

This will happen. It will happen because people want to live.

Dr. Attia:

If I were gonna give you one suggestion, it would be: Do this from a position of pull, not push.

So right now, you are pushing this idea. What you really want to do is take a page out of the Charlie Foundation, where they're basically saying:

„Look, in the end the results were so dramatic that the parents of the children - a third of whom now no longer suffer from epilepsy, another third of whom have at least a 50% reduction in epilepsy...." Those parents basically became the voice of reason.

I think the data were good in epilepsy. But I think that the parents and their advicacy were the main reason why today, the

219

only place where a ketogenic diet is viewed as a legitimate first-line therapy for recalcitrant disease, is in epilepsy!

I think there will be a day when that expands to other disease as well, like cancer.

What I would hope is that there's a network of people, family members probably, who have lost people to GBM, would become the ones that would be your mouthpiece, right?

Would become the ones that would say

„You know what? I'm tired of the fact that my loved one died in 9 months, seemingly in vain, and there's this body of evidence that maybe could have helped.

That body of evidence is admittedly small and uncertain at this point is, but nothing in science is certain.

But: They're offering an alternative. I want to know that that could be tested."

Prof. Seyfried:
The thing that kills me with these private foundations is: Their advisory boards are made up of physicians that subscribe to the gene theory of cancer. So when the patients and their advocates hear about this...

(...)

Dr. Attia:
I think metabolic therapies could be valuable whether or not the genetic ideas of cancer are right or wrong.

(...)

Anyway, on that note I want to thank you very much for your generosity of time - and just your passion for this and and how tirelessly you've worked on this.

Is there anything that someone who's listening to this, who's got a loved one who's either died of GBM or has GBM...

What can they do to increase the chances that either others can get the types of therapies you're talking about in clinical trials, or that their loved ones themselves can?

What else can we do?

Prof. Seyfried:
I mean, in my position as a researcher who does the preclinical studies, we get support from Travis foundation, the Metabolic Therapy Foundation - and that's what keeps our program going. That's what tells us what we think should work really well or

what might not work to help these people get the outcome that they want. Which is high quality of life and living a lot longer.

My big thing is that, we can identify those strategies. And you need funds for that. The federal government is mostly like what gene is involved? So this is where it comes back to the same problem again: You don't get funding for things that actually can really work versus studying the disease.

„Let's study the disease more" - we don't need to study it more, we have a path.

Dr. Attia:
Is there an easy path for patients who want to make financial contributions to the lab? Is it through a foundation?

Prof. Seyfried:
Yes, there's two ways to do it. You could either do it through the Foundation, because we have a continual grant set up through the *Single Cause Single Cure Foundation.*

And also at Boston College. If you want to fund the work directly through the University. It has to be through a very specific statement, otherwise the university will absorb it.

What we do then is: We give our data immediately to the clinical people, who then put it on their patients - and then feed me back and say this is working well or we don't think this is doing as well as we wanted.

You tweak it in this or that direction after that feedack. So I work with the physicians directly and I give them the preclinical information, they feed me back and see how it's working.

Sometimes it works a hell of a lot better in the human than in the mouse!

Dr. Attia:
Maybe the relatives of diseased or sick loved ones will create a bit of a groundswell, that puts a little bit of pressure on the IRBs to say Look, GBM is as high-stakes as it gets... Right? It's the type of cancer that gives cancer a bad name.

And maybe this is one area where we have to increase our appetite for risk in clinical trials.

Prof. Seyfried:
I agree with that. I think that this is a disease that we can make major advances in, and why not want to give it a shot? Because it's not going to hurt anybody, it's not gonna accelerate their demise.

(...)

This has been really exciting and I really appreciate your time and your insights. And above all else, the work you've done! So thanks Tom!

Prof. Seyfried:

Thank you!

Chapter 6: The Origin (and future) of the Ketogenic Diet

In the front yard, on an innocent spring morning in 1993, Hollywood movie producer, Jim Abrahams, rhythmically pushed his son Charlie in a swing. Behind him were the busy noises of his wife Nancy and Charlie's two siblings as they prepared the house for a celebration – it was Charlie's first birthday.

Nobody was prepared for what came next. It happened in a moment. Suddenly Charlie's head slumped to the side, and then out of nowhere his arm shot into the air, as if possessed by some unseen force. Deep down Abrahams knew that something was seriously wrong. A moment before his son was healthy, and now, a fleeting instant later, he was not.

A series of neurological tests proved his instincts were correct. "Your son has epilepsy," the neurologist told him. He then went on to explain that epilepsy, although a single diagnosis, really consists of a wide spectrum of illness; from mild to severe, and within the spectrum the seizures that define the disease are as diverse as a box of crayons. Partial, generalized, and absence seizures comprise the three main groupings.

These are then further parsed into tonic, clonic, tonic-clonic, myoclonic, and atonic seizures. Each category describes a choreographed path of involuntary muscle contractions that spin outward from the neurological chaos unraveling within the brain.

As some time passed, tragically, Charlie's case landed more toward the severe end of the spectrum, and it wasn't just the nature of the seizures, it was the frequency – he was having up to one-hundred seizures a day. It was heartbreaking to watch. Time after time the toddler's brain was taken over while he tried to play. In the middle of stacking a block, or blowing a horn, he would pause, and then slump over, sometimes remaining still, and others with a limb or two shaking uncontrollably. And then it was over, and life would more or less resume where it left off.

It was life lived in intervals. A day was not the seamless continuum most of us take for granted, it was a chopped up into tiny little slices. "It was a fate worse than death," said Abrahams. "The house was filled with tears, all of us, all the time, cried."

Charlie was put on one medication after another – a process that seemed haphazard and experimental. The odds were already stacked against them. If an epileptic child fails the first drug, the chance the next drug will work drops to 10 to 15 percent. Nevertheless, the doses were upped, and the drugs were given in combination; new with old, old with new, but nothing seemed to blunt the attacks.

Worse, the Abrahamses watched helplessly as the drugs changed their child in the few good moments he was spared. "You pour the drugs down your child's throat despite the fact there is something inside you that says, 'wait a minute this can't be right'", said Abrahams. "My son was so loaded at times he just lived in his car seat....he was essentially nonfunctional."

The Abrahamses were delicately told by the doctors that Charlie's illness came with additional consequences. The severity and frequency, at this age, would affect the development of his brain – if left unchecked, it would lead to progressive retardation. So it was a race against time. Desperate, the Abrahamses did everything they could. The physician they went to at UCLA, Dr. Donald Shields, was a nationally recognized expert in children's epilepsy. They didn't stop there. They sought a second, third, fourth, and fifth opinion. But nothing new was offered, each doctors opinion was just a reiteration of the last: stick with the drugs. But the drugs simply weren't working.

The doctors didn't seem to share the Abrahamses sense of urgency. Every day was important; Charlie was slowly falling into an abyss. The doctors finally capitulated, and they turned to the option held in reserve: surgery. But the glimmer of hope surgery held vanished once Charlie recovered and the relentless assault of seizures continued. With nowhere left to turn, at the end of the road, the Abrahamses turned to a faith healer. Still nothing.

For the Abrahamses, if any sort of resignation creeped in, it only served to stoke a fire. There is no greater instinctual surge than of protective parents. "After thousands of epileptic seizures, an incredible number of drugs, dozens of blood draws, eight hospitalizations, a mountain of EEG's, MRI's, CT scans and PET scans, one fruitless brain surgery, five pediatric neurologists in three cities, two homeopaths, one faith healer, and countless prayers, the seizures continued unchecked.." But giving up was never an option.

And so Jim Abrahams began his own research. He began combing through books and attending medical lectures. It was an education rolled up in a frantic mission. Then one day, on the bottom shelve at the medical library, he picked up a book published that year by Dr. John Freeman, titled *Seizures and Epilepsy in Childhood: A Guide for Parents*. The book was written for parents to help them cope. But buried deep inside were three pages on a dietary protocol used to treat epilepsy. Dr. Freeman had tried to write a book focused solely on the diet but was unable to find a publisher – so he snuck them into this book almost as an afterthought.

Within the few pages was the remarkable claim that the diet was able to help at least half of those who maintained it. The first impulse that ran through Abrahams mind was bewilderment. If it had *any* legitimacy, why hadn't one of the five doctors mentioned this treatment option by now? "I couldn't make the leap between all these doctors saying one thing and this other guy saying something else," he later confessed. Confused and desperate, he had what he felt were only two options left: the strange diet, and an herbalist someone had told him about working out of a strip mall in Houston Texas.

At the next appointment, when he asked Dr. Shields which one he should pursue, Shields said, "Flip a coin, neither will probably work." And so he did just that, he and his wife Nancy literally flipped a coin: heads the herbalist, tails the strange diet. It landed on heads. The family traveled to Houston and met the herbalist. They took his advice, bought a grocery bag full of herbs, and returned home. After a few weeks of mixing herbal teas it became apparent the strange smelling concoctions were having no effect on Charlie's seizures.

This was the end of the line. The best doctors in the world, the best drugs in the world, surgery, homeopaths, faith healers, herbalists, everything had failed Charlie. Charlie and his family were backed into a corner. There was only one option left. So, with only a thread of hope; desperate, deflated, and exhausted, the Abrahamses boarded a plane to Baltimore Maryland to see John Freeman about the peculiar and obscure treatment called *the ketogenic diet.*

Oddly enough, as they flew to the east coast, at some point in the upper Midwest, perhaps over the Ohio Valley, if the

Abrahamses could have peered eighty years into the past, they would have looked down and seen a train heading in the opposite direction to Battle Creek Michigan. On board were their exact counterparts: a desperate family with their epileptic son, at the end of their rope, traveling to the only option left to them – a long shot.

Mark Twain said "history doesn't repeat itself, but it does rhyme." And the stories of these families rhymed in every sentence and verse. But in a larger context, each story, astonishing in its own right, serve only as bookmarks: it is what happened in the interim, the eighty years that lie in-between, which reveals volumes. Critically, it is a vitally important lesson of the infallibility and undulating path of medical science, and a stark reminder that valuable knowledge, even in the modern era, can be lost.

––––––––

The story of both families converge on a single man: Bernard Macfadden. Although almost entirely forgotten today, in the early 1900's almost everyone knew his name. Macfadden was a bona fide American icon. His rise to fame was also uniquely American, he started with nothing. In fact, less than nothing; he was cast into the world with the odds decidedly stacked against him. His early years were filled with pain and abandonment. His father beat him and his family before drinking himself to death when Macfadden was five years old.

When Macfadden was seven, his mother sent him away to the cheapest boarding school she could find because she was dying from late-stage tuberculosis and was unable to care for him any longer. Macfadden then escaped what he called the "starvation school" and fell into a series of indentured servitudes for distant relatives and farmers, working one-hundred hour weeks and paid only in room and board.

But like all American icons Macfadden fought back, scratching and clawing for a better place in the world. When he was fifteen he accidentally wandered into a newly established gymnasium in St. Louis. One look past the threshold was all it took. Inside men were grunting and sweating while they hoisting dumbbells and preformed calisthenics, posters of musclemen plastered the walls. As he stared open-mouthed and wide-eyed Macfadden was at the same time enthralled and infected. Right there he swore an oath: "I'm going to look like them, I'm going to be like them."

Over time, Macfadden parlayed his sworn oath into an empire. Recognizing an opportunity, he started a magazine called *Physical Culture*. What started as a modest enterprise soon rocketed skyward with dazzling growth. It was a fresh, new message for Americans. Within the pages he proselytized health, vitality, and uninhibited enjoyment of the human body. He advocated exercise, healthy eating, and avoidance of tobacco, too much alcohol, and white bread (a substance Macfadden called the "staff of death").

He encouraged nude sunbathing, walking barefoot, and warned of the evils of prudishness – the body, claimed Macfadden, was for unrestrained enjoyment. For the first time Americans were told sex was good, and was nothing to be ashamed of. His magazines were provocative (the first to use scantily clad models); engaging, and told American's there was a new and better way to live.

He had tapped into a new niche, he had become America's first health guru, forging a new culture and selling a lifestyle. He was the driving force behind the rise of body-building. He hand-picked an unknown Brooklyn model named Charles Atlas and gave him the title "World's Most Perfect Man", and then was the architect behind a career path that led to Atlas's fame and fortune.

American's appetite for Macfadden's new lifestyle was insatiable. Half way through the year 1900, Macfadden was selling 110,000 copies of *Physical Culture* per month. His rapid success came with a new cockiness. The wildly popular magazine, claimed Macfadden, not only blazed the path to health and vitality, now, it was revealing his secrets to curing disease – *any disease*. His belief was sincere, and consisted of a prescriptive life style that he claimed would bring anyone back from the throes of illness.

The prescription consisted of the principles he had been proselytizing for most of his life: exercise, sunlight, avoidance of alcohol, tobacco, and diet. But the most important piece, the one imperative ingredient to pull people from the ghostly realm of the sick back into vitality, was something Macfadden felt held almost magical healing properties: *fasting.*

Macfadden's belief in fasting, while maybe largely forgotten, certainly wasn't new. Its restorative powers go far back into antiquity. The Greek physician, Hippocrates, made reference to the healing properties of fasting, "Everyone has a doctor in him; we just have to help him in his work. The natural healing force within each one of us is the greatest force in getting well. ...to eat when you are sick, is to feed your sickness." Incredibly, the virtues of fasting, or overconsumption in general, went even further back, all the way to 3800BC. An inscription found in an Egyptian pyramid read:

"Humans live on one-quarter of what they eat; on the other three-quarters lives their doctor." (A glib quote that could easily describe the relationship between food and medicine today). Other famous people have touted fasting throughout history, including Ben Franklin, "The best of all medicines is resting and fasting." Mark Twain wrote, "A little starvation can really do more for the average sick man than can the best medicines and the best doctors."

Macfadden embraced the time honored practice that had strangely bounced in and out of favor through thousands of years of history. Perhaps the counterintuitive nature of sick people not eating served to pull it back into obscurity time and time again. Rarely would a grandmother, parent, or a physician in their right mind suggest that a sick person should stop eating – it goes against every fiber of instinct.

However Macfadden stumbled onto the salubrious practice of fasting, his faith in its powers were reinforced by personal observation and trial. While working on a farm, he had noticed that whenever an animal became ill it stopped eating. Years later, one spring he felt the early symptoms of pneumonia stirring in his chest. He remembered the lesson of the farm animals and cut back to a couple pieces of fruit per day. He noticed by the second day his chest had begun to clear and by the fourth day the symptoms had all but vanished.

Macfadden's sideways entry into medicine ultimately culminated in the creation of a sanatorium in 1907 – a massive mansion equipped with swimming pools, gyms, Russian and Turkish baths, and relaxation areas. The Bernarr Macfadden Sanatorium (he had changed his name from Bernard to Bernarr because it sounded like the roar of a lion) was located in Battle

Creek Michigan, a small town turned overnight into a beacon for the sick. Directly across the street stood the famous Battle Creek Sanitarium, started by John Harvey Kellogg (his brother capitalized on the health trend and started the Kellogg cereal company).

Three hundred thousand health seekers visited the Battle Creek Sanitarium during its 65 years of operation. Every day the train dropped off a fresh crop complaining of a variety of ailments — a portion of which now headed to Macfadden's new sanatorium with the hope of getting well. Most of those that showed up on Macfadden's doorstep had vague symptoms like headaches, weight loss, digestive problems, and it was really no surprise, the typical diet of a century ago consisted mostly of salt pork, bread, and potatoes.

The first vitamin would not be discovered until 1912 and American's were entirely unaware how deficient their diets truly were. Also, the workforce had begun the transition to desk jobs. The combination of a terrible diet and inactivity left many Americans in a sorry state – they turned to Macfadden to help.

At the sanatorium Macfadden hired an osteopath doctor named Hugh Conklin as an assistant. He prescribed to the same belief system as Macfadden. They both believed that medicine, the way it was practiced, was largely fraudulent. Together they called out the medical establishment: *we will take those you have given up on and cure them.* This was fine for the mostly vague and un-diagnosable masses that showed up. After a period of stress free fasting, hydrotherapy, and light exercise in and around the beautiful mansion they did feel better.

Of course, some of the more conservative doctors pushed back, claiming Macfadden and his hand-picked doctors were the worst kind of quacks: "the kind that preyed on those that were healthy but thought they were sick." But Macfadden had star power on his side. Of his more famous clients, Upton Sinclair, defended him vigorously, even publishing a book *titled The Fasting Cure,* dedicated to his good friend B.M.

Occasionally patients with very tangible illnesses, like epilepsy, showed up on Macfadden's doorstep. For the detractors of McFadden, this, they thought, would surely be where he would fail. Epileptic patients, in particular, came with a built-in yardstick. The therapies prescribed would face a true test

229

because of one simple fact: the number of seizures could be counted before and after treatment, thus determining if treatment was effective or not.

It's not clear if Conklin or Macfadden knew the history of epilepsy. If they did, they would have known there was a scattering of evidence backing the idea fasting would work for epilepsy. In the fifth century BC, Hippocrates reported on a man who had been seized by convulsions. A fast was prescribed and the cure worked, freeing the individual of seizures. In a quotation from the King James Version of the Bible, Mark tells the story of Jesus curing an epileptic boy where his disciples had failed. When they asked him why, Jesus said, "this kind can come out by nothing but prayer and fasting."

And so Conklin began to count. He recorded the number of seizures before and after treatment. When the numbers were tallied the result was shocking and undeniable: *fasting worked for epileptic patients.* Once they stopped eating an invisible metabolic levy was raised around the brain. The neurological storms that once pounded the shores were abruptly dispelled. For some reason, however, Conklin felt no immediate compulsion to publish his data. But it didn't matter. Nature abhors a vacuum – the medical establishment had no good solutions – and so word of the "drugless healer" in Battle Creek, Michigan claiming to have an effective treatment for epilepsy, gradually began filtering into the public at large.

As rumors of Conklin's "water diet" rippled outward from the center of the country, doctors continued to treat epilepsy with the few drugs they had. The most commonly prescribed drug was potassium bromide. In the mid 1800's it was thought epilepsy was caused by excessive sexual indulgence and particularly masturbation. In 1857, a British doctor, Charles Lockhart, read a report claiming people had become temporarily impotent after taking potassium bromide. By his own reckoning, Lockhart made the connection: maybe the drug would assuage the sexual gluttony of epileptics, and as a result, stop their seizures? The drug worked in spite of Lockhart's faulty logic.

A decade later doctors began questioning the link between excessive sexuality and epilepsy. More likely, they reasoned, Bromide was acting directly on the brain rather than through the indirect suppression of sexual desire. Bromide is a powerful

230

sedative, and researchers made the irresistible connection between the nervous eruption of a seizure and the drugs ability to slow nervous impulses – like pouring water on a fire. In 1872 one researcher wrote, "The object of medical treatment for epilepsy is to control the over-readyness of nervous action.

For this purpose sedatives have been employed with success." The connection was powerfully seductive, and would guide the search for new anti-seizure medications for the foreseeable future. The search for new epilepsy drugs was now synonymous to finding drugs that were sedative – the two qualities were thought to be inseparable.

The next breakthrough happened on a fall day in 1912. It happened because a young medical student named Alfred Hauptman was sleep deprived. The young German, resident-psychiatrist, lived over the epileptic ward while he was in medical training. Below him, seizures tormented his patients throughout the night. He could hear them thrash and convulse, sometimes even the thud of one of them falling out of bed. The unremitting sounds forbade sleep. As he tossed and turned he realized he had to try something. A new sleeping pill called Luminal had just hit the pharmacy a year earlier.

During his medical training he learned potassium bromide worked as an anti-seizure medication precisely because it was a sedative. It wasn't unreasonable to think that Luminal might work through the same mechanism. In the very least, he thought, maybe both he and his patients could get a good night's sleep. And so the next evening, right before bedtime, he gave each of his patients a dose of the new drug. To his delight, Hauptmann slept soundly that night, as did his patients. He would have left it at that, a simple remedy for a good night sleep, but he noticed something remarkable: his patient's reprieve from seizures extended into the next day – *they didn't have any.*

Hauptmann made the connection hovering before him: perhaps this drug, chemically known as phenobarbital, could be a new medication for epilepsy. Once he published his observation phenobarbital began to be prescribed and slowly built momentum, eventually overtaking potassium bromide's position as the first line treatment for epilepsy. Although better at preventing seizures than potassium bromide, for patients, Luminal was still a compromise – fewer seizures was swapped for a life lived in a fog – a hazy, blunted state of existence. Doctor's assumed it was a zero sum game – fewer seizures came at the expense of sedation. It was accepted this was just the way it had to be.

Charles Howland's Question

In 1921, H. Rawle Geyelin, a prominent endocrinologist at New York Presbyterian Hospital, took the podium at the annual American Medical Association convention. Rather than the typical, dry run through mountains of graphs and charts, Geyelin chose to tell a story. He spoke of a young cousin who had epilepsy. Over four years he watched as his cousin tried every treatment recommended by several neurologists, including the boy's uncle who was a professor of pediatrics at Johns Hopkins. The family watched helpless as every treatment failed, including bromides and the newer drug phenobarbital (Luminal). The desperate family took what they saw as the only option left: a train ride to Battle Creek Michigan to see Macfadden and Conklin.

By now Conklin had treated an untold number of patients, probably numbering in the hundreds. Geyelin explained how the young cousin fasted under the supervision of Conklin for three or four weeks. Remarkably, the seizures stopped after the second day, and the remission proved remarkably durable – his cousin remained seizure free for over two years after completion of the treatment.

For Geyelin, it was impossible to ignore the result. First, because of the intimate family connection, and second because he knew his cousin had failed every other treatment, the best those in the audience – the doctors sitting before him – had to offer. So Geyelin looked closer. He carefully followed two other patients that traveled to Battle Creek to see Dr. Conklin. The patients, Geyelin confirmed, at least for the time being, were cured – they remained free of seizures after returning home.

Geyelin then took the next logical step. He saw if he could replicate Conklin's results by fasting his own patients. Now, in front of the hushed audience, he presented the results. After fasting 30 patients for 20 days in his clinic: 87% of the patients became seizure free. The results evoked gasps from the audience. The rumors of the drugless Midwestern healer that publicly announce his disdain for conventional medicine were now staring them in the face. It was no longer a rumor; Geyelin had cast it into documented fact.

For the doctors in the auditorium, the treatment of epilepsy remained as frustrating of an enterprise as it always had. "Surely patients with no other disease have grasped at so many therapeutic straws," wrote one doctor. Epilepsy comes from Ancient Greece meaning "to seize, posses, or afflict". The Greeks also called epilepsy the sacred disease, and as civilizations before them, they thought it was a form of spiritual possession.

Consequently, for century's, victims were treated with one pointless ritual after the next. In the fifth century B.C. Hippocrates boldly challenged the assumption epilepsy was divine in origin declaring it was a medically treatable problem emanating from the brain. Hippocrates' declaration would change the course of the disease forever, thrusting it into the empirical arena of real medicine.

But the transition would not be smooth. His declaration started what would be a series of clumsy, barbaric, and sometimes bizarre attempts to treat the disease. The eccentric and unrelated treatments were a reflection of the fact epilepsy was of mysterious and unknown origin. Doctor's attempts to mute epileptic fits were patchwork of trial and error: bloodletting, trephining of the skull (boring a hole in the skull to release the disease), removal of the ovaries and adrenal glands, countless drugs, herbs, and tinctures.

When the Roman physician Celsus witnessed epileptics drinking blood from the wounds of dying gladiators he wrote: "What a miserable disease that makes tolerable such a miserable remedy." And in 1921, as Geyelin gave his presentation, little had changed. "Many Modern 'cures' are not less miserable" wrote a respected neurologist, comparing the state of treatment in the 1920's to those of the past. Doctors still had little to offer the victims of epilepsy; and that a nonconventional osteopath had discovered what might be the best treatment available was met with a degree of skepticism, frustration, and embarrassment.

The father of Geyelin's young cousin, Charles Howland, was a wealthy New York corporate attorney. Shocked that the cure to his son's epilepsy lie so far outside the medical establishment, Howland became obsessed with a single question: *why did fasting cure his son of epilepsy?* Conklin already thought he knew the answer. He claimed epilepsy emanated from the intestines. He speculated that toxins were secreted from the lymph nodes surrounding the small intestine then stored in the lymph system, and from time to time, discharged into the bloodstream, causing seizures. Simply not eating allowed the toxins to be cleared.

Conklin had no evidence to back his claim; his reasoning was nothing more than a wild guess, probably pushed along by Macfadden. Along with many doctors, Charles Howland wasn't satisfied with Conklin's contrived explanation. Instinctually, Howland felt there was more to it. He desperately wanted to know – he wanted an answer backed by actual evidence. In hope of finding an answer, he wrote a check to his brother, a professor of Pediatrics at Johns Hopkins, for five-thousand dollars.

Five thousand dollars went a long way in the early 1900's and Dr. Howland used the money to set up a state of the art laboratory at Johns Hopkins dedicated to the new mission. As with his brother, the question quickly became a particular obsession. The answer, reasoned Howland, was sure to lie within some shift in the epileptic's metabolism. To find the answer would be an exercise in comparison. What did the metabolism of the epileptic look like before and after fasting, and could the relevant factor be isolated from the noise? Far too steep a task for any individual, he turned to Dr. James Gamble, an unusually precise and methodical clinical chemist.

The canvas for Gamble's search consisted of four fasting epileptic children. He carefully monitored every known biochemical variable as they transitioned into the fasting state. He collected and exhaustively analyzed their urine and blood with painstaking detail – from water loss, to electrolytes balance, acid/base balance, and the curious mention of the strange occurrence of two ketones, *beta hydroxybutyrate and acetoacetate*, in the fasting patient's plasma and urine. To Gamble, the compounds were a mystery. He speculated that they were meaningless; the byproduct of the "incomplete oxidation of fats" – nothing more than a useless exhaust expelled as the patients began to burn fat.

In the end, despite an extensive search, the report held no definitive answer, the biochemical shift that reduced seizures in fasting epileptics, for the time being, remained a mystery. As Howland's team continued its frenzied search, about a thousand miles west, in Chicago, the seeds were being planted to offer up a different explanation.

Food Becomes Medicine

Rowland Woodyatt and Evarts Graham, both medical doctors in Chicago, were having an argument over lunch. The waiter was already tense. Their voices were elevated and, worse, they had scribbled arcane symbols all over the table cloth, it was most likely ruined. The argument had drifted away from the scribblings into something more personal. "Your perfectionism is holding you back, can't you see that," said Graham, clearly frustrated. "Did you know it took Lorenzo Ghiberti twenty years just to sculpt the bronze doors of the baptistery of San Giovanni. Perfection doesn't care how long something takes," retorted Woodyatt, in a measured voice. Woodyatt was a perfectionist, in every sense of the word, and Graham was not the first to notice.

He could agonize over the wording of a single sentence, sometimes for an entire day. Graham found this absurd, a waste of time and talent. But for the study of human metabolism, Woodyatt's peculiar personality trait was perhaps his greatest strength. He was intensely passionate about the details. He could zero in, focus with singular purpose, and not allow himself to be railroaded by the incredibly complex maze of metabolic pathways where others quickly became overwhelmed.

In the summer of 1921, Woodyatt's passion for metabolism culminated in an article titled: *Objects and Method of Diet Adjustment in Diabetes*. Although insulin had yet to be isolated, researchers knew that the pancreas was the site of pathology – injecting diabetic dogs with pancreatic extract could normalize blood sugar levels. Woodyatt realized that the problem in the diabetic lie solely in pancreatic dysfunction, resulting in an inability to utilize excessive carbohydrate. At the time, physician's often fasted diabetics until glucose disappeared from the urine, the idea being to "rest" the pancreas. A normal diet was then slowly reintroduced, usually with carbohydrates first. Unfortunately, the diabetics soon found themselves back where they started, with sugar building up to malevolent levels within the blood stream.

That fasting cleared the bloodstream of sugar made Woodyatt curious, inspiring him to ask a simple question: if fasting diabetic patients resort to burning their own fat, why not just provide fat through diet, keep the carbohydrates away, and keep the diabetic in the fasted state indefinitely? It was a simple proposal of exclusion. It was a question that perhaps should have been asked sooner, but at the time it was easy for researchers to get lost in the details. Big questions still lingered, the largest was the fate of dietary fat: it was not clear if fat could be converted directly into sugar. But Woodyatt refused to let the gaps in knowledge lead to a dead end – when a pathway was unknown, he let empirical, macro-evidence guide him.

In this case, he knew another group had already experimented with a high fat/low carb diet in diabetics with striking success – even if fat was able to be converted into glucose it really didn't matter, reasoned Woodyatt, something appeared to be blocking its conversion. He was formulating a hypothesis that had only lingered in and out of researcher's minds, but had never been concretely suggested.

Once he wrote it down, it seemed obvious: *why not shift the ratio of the diet in favor of fat, this way the diabetic would be able to rest his pancreas, remove the excess sugar from his bloodstream, and utilize fat instead as an energy source.* The smoldering problems of insulin, carbohydrates, and blood sugar were removed from the equation.

He couldn't help chastising the medical community for their inflexible, dogmatic assumptions, isolating the problem as a tendency toward dietary groupthink: "the universal custom of thinking of the food supply simply as so much carbohydrate, so much protein, so much fat and so many calories without further analysis," wrote Woodyatt. The patient doesn't even have to be deprived, he reasoned, they could consume the same amount of total calories. In a single sentence Woodyatt toppled the monolithic view of diet. Now, because of him, diet was no longer viewed as a concrete pillar, now it was a column built from subcategories (carbohydrate, protein, and fat) that could be manipulated, shifted, and restacked in different combinations depending on the needs of the patient.

While Woodyatt was exposing fissures in dietary preconceptions, in the summer of 1921, three hundred and fifty miles north east of Chicago at the Mayo clinic in Rochester Minnesota, a doctor named Russell Wilder published three short paragraphs in *The Clinical Bulletin*. The letter described the same dietary epiphany as Woodyatt — maintaining the fasting state by replacing carbohydrates with fat – but Wilder imagined treating a different disease: epilepsy. "It has occurred to us that the benefit of Dr. Geyelin's procedure may be dependent on the ketonemia which must result from such fasts, and that possibly equally good results could be obtained if a ketonemia were produced by some other means," wrote Wilder. But Wilder had made an additional leap of logic.

Woodyatt had suggested the dietary protocol simply as a means to sidestep the impaired carbohydrate metabolism of diabetics. How fasting, or the dietary maintenance of fasting, worked to control seizures demanded another explanation. Wilder reasoned perhaps there was more to it – suggesting the ketones generated from the diet might be of unrecognized significance.

After all, they were the single metabolic variable shared between the fasting state and a low/carb high/fat diet. Until now, researchers assumed ketones were nothing but unhealthy metabolic debris, but now, because of Wilder, that assumption was questioned. Perhaps it was ketones themselves that were pulling the metabolic levers inside the brain of fasting epileptics. Wilder was anxious to test his theory. "It is proposed, therefore, to try the effect of such *ketogenic diets* on a series of epileptics."

It's hard to quantify the influence that words have. Attaching a name to an idea converts it from an abstraction into something tangible and concrete. Wilder's naming of the "ketogenic diet" was to thrust it into the clinic, now it was real, now it was something that could be measured, tested, and prescribed.

Under the lamp of Woodyatt and Wilder's clarifying epiphanies, Dr. Mynie Peterman, a mayo clinic pediatrician, enthusiastically put Wilder's theoretical diet to a clinical test. First, he strictly defined the ketogenic diet to be tested, parceling it into one gram of protein per kilogram of the child's body weight, 10-15 grams of carbohydrates per day, and the remainder of the calories in fat. Next, he began recruiting epileptic patients and convincing them to try the strange protocol.

The scientific community was watching closely – they eagerly waited for the results. Once released, Peterman's report revealed the diet's effect was incredible. Most of the children, once racked with convulsions, experienced an immediate and powerful remission. They began to live normal lives. The price was minimal. Occasional a child became nauseated and vomited, and so Peterman found a little orange juice was an instant fix. But most transitioned to the new diet well and had few complaints.

The ketogenic diet, at first only a fragile theory, was working. While running his clinical trials Peterman noticed something else. Not only were the vast majority of kids either experiencing greatly diminished numbers of seizures, or free of them altogether, but there seemed to be a striking change in their character. Peterman noticed the children were "sleeping better, were less irritable, and displayed an increased interest and alertness." This was in sharp contrast to the pharmacological treatments that dulled and muted the children, as if a wet blanket was pulled over their brains.

The ketogenic diet, Peterman observed, lifted the fog. Peterman followed 37 children on the diet for 4 months up to two and a half years. All tallied, sixty percent of the children became seizure free, 34.5% were improved, and 5.5% were not improved. The ketogenic diet was a resounding success – undeniably better than phenobarbital and bromides.

While the newly débuted "ketogenic diet" was being studied at the Mayo clinic, doctors on the East coast were still deeply immersed in neurochemical transformation induced by fasting. Therapeutically, fasting had obvious limitations. The biggest problem, doctors realized, is that fasting was clearly only a temporary solution. The seizures were greatly diminished, if not stopped altogether while the child was not eating, but of course, it could not be maintained. In some of the more mild cases, after the fast, the seizures never returned. But in many cases, once the child resumed eating, the seizures gradually resumed. Wilder's ketogenic diet offered an immediate solution to this problem. The therapeutic effect of fasting could now be extended on a patient by patient basis.

News from the Mayo clinic trial quickly spread. Massachusetts General Hospital, in 1924, pivoted away from fasting and adopted the ketogenic diet as a treatment for epilepsy. Others were soon to follow. New studies tallied similar results as the original done by Peterman, and others also noticed the positive effects the diet seemed to have on the children, one researcher commented, "the diet is well tolerated without causing any untoward symptoms in the patients. On the contrary, they seem to be more alert and less nervous." After tinkering with the ratios, clinicians determined that a formula of 4 parts fat to 1 part protein/carbohydrate seemed to work best (a ratio that has stood the test of time and today is known as the *classic ketogenic diet*.)

Instructions for the ketogenic diet, meal plans, and extensive tables listing the nutritional composition of foods were added to textbooks. In response to rising demand, the Mayo Clinic published a pamphlet describing detailed meal plans and recipes for the ketogenic diet. Soon clinicians and dietitians at hospitals across the county were prescribing the new dietary treatment for epilepsy.

Untold numbers of families with epileptic children were restocking their pantries and adjusting their family dinners. For doctors, and the families of the afflicted, it was probably an easy choice, the only two drugs on the market were highly sedative, and the diet was the opposite; it required some work, it wasn't an easy fix, but the benefit was striking, immediate, and enduring for most. Word swiftly spread and the ketogenic diet became the preferred therapy for epilepsy across the country. "The results of fasting and the ketogenic diet are apparently the best that are obtained by any therapeutic procedure that we have to offer the epileptics in childhood today," Geyelin told the American College of Physicians at a gathering in New Orleans in 1928.

"Like Stones for a Mosaic"

Charles Howland refused to give up. In 1922, undeterred by his brother and Gamble's failure to find a definitive answer, he set out to expand the list of experts to help answer his question. He singled out Dr. Stanley Cobb, the associate professor of neuropathology at Harvard Medical School. Cobb was a cautious and careful scientist from a prominent Boston family that was speculated to have entered the neurosciences as a result of a childhood stammer. Cobb was already familiar with Howland's story – he was in the audience a year earlier when Geyelin presented the case of his young cousin's trek to Battle Creek and the successful treatment by Conklin.

To Cobb, the story was not entirely surprising. Rumors of Conklin's early results had intrigued him, and he had begun to investigate fasting's effect within his own lab. When Geyelin had finished his presentation, Cobb excitedly shared his own work with the attendees, commenting that he had witnessed the therapeutic effect first-hand – preventing convulsions in animals by fasting them.

What *did* surprise Cobb, however, was that now, one year later, the father of the child Geyelin spoke of was standing in his office, and asking for his help. Cobb had revealed how he felt about Conklin's work in an earlier conversation with a colleague when he stated that fasting treatment was significant because it "revealed the relationship between epilepsy and metabolism." In Cobb's mind, this relationship demanded to be explored. Cobb agreed to help. Howland scribbled out a check for enough to fund Cobb's efforts for two years.

Cobb knew the difficulty of what he had just signed up for. He would have to tap the same dogged grit that allowed him to overcome his childhood stammer. To get to the bottom of Howland's question was to step into the unknown – despite Gamble's intense effort, few solid leads had been found – all that was known for sure was fasting worked. Instinctually, he knew he would need help.

First on Cobb's list to conscript into the effort was a Harvard educated doctor named William Lennox. Enthusiastic, innovative, and bold, Lennox became interested in epilepsy after witnessing the unrelenting and mysterious convulsions of a friend's daughter while studying the health of missionary families in China in 1917. The strange nature of the disease stirred something in Lennox. In a stroke of serendipity, Lennox happened to be visiting Boston in the spring of 1921 and attended the AMA meeting where Geyelin presented. Suddenly, Lennox found himself at a turning point. He commented that he was "thrilled by Geyelin's demonstration and having a compelling interest in epilepsy and its treatment, my missionary zeal was abruptly transferred from Chinese to epilepsy," The timing was perfect – infused with Howland's cash, Cobb offered Lennox a position. It didn't take much convincing from Cobb to recruit Lennox. The intense curiosity simmering inside him made the decision easy.

Together they launched into the problem. Howland's question was now expanded to include the ketogenic diet that had been defined a year earlier by Wilder. The diet was the preservation of the fasting state, and so by extension, the same rules probably applied. Whatever mechanism fasting worked through to mitigate seizures was most likely the same for the ketogenic diet. Wilder had added another suspect to the lineup: ketone bodies. Like Gamble, Cobb and Lennox dove into the metabolic transformation that occurred within fasting epileptic patients with painstaking detail. And like Gamble, after some time had passed, they realized the answer was not going to present itself easily. Strangely, it seemed every path they followed ended with a contradiction – as if they were purposefully being toyed with.

For example, Geyelin had noticed his fasting patients excreted acid – the more acid excreted, the fewer seizures. Ketones are acidic, so maybe, they reasoned, it was the increase in acidosis within the patient's blood plasma from ketosis that was somehow acting to slow seizures. Other clues led them in this direction. Acidifying the patient's plasma by injecting acid directly into their veins seemed to have an anti-seizure effect. But the problem was in the timing.

The anti-seizure effect didn't exactly track the acidification – once the pH level was made acidic, it took a while for the seizures to slow. Similarly, when the blood pH level was returned to normal, it took some time for the seizures to return. This didn't match with the fact the induction of ketosis, either by fasting or the ketogenic diet, typically resulted in an immediate reduction in seizures – so clearly it wasn't the acidity alone that mattered. Also, when they acidified the patients' blood, their seizures eventually slowed, but then after a period of time, even while the blood was kept acidic, the seizures would roar back with vicious ferocity, as if a damn had been burst.

Maybe, as Wilder suggested, it was the ketone bodies themselves? To test this idea Lennox and Cobb put a patient on the ketogenic diet. Once her seizures stopped, she was injected with bi-carbonate (a compound that counteracts acid). When they tested her blood after the injection of bi-carbonate, surprisingly, there was an increase in ketone bodies, but, even with the increased ketones, her seizures returned with a vengeance – so clearly it wasn't the ketone bodies by themselves. Every time they tried to isolate the relevant variable it would slip just out of reach.

The nature of the problem was not lost on Cobb and Lennox. They recognized what it was: an incredibly complex and interrelated series of neurochemical alterations. The search, they realized, was probably just getting started: "The painstaking accumulation of apparently unrelated facts must go on," wrote Lennox, "until, like stones for a mosaic, they are sufficient in number to permit their assembly into a complete and intelligible design." The answer remained a map of the world before Columbus. The yet-to-be-explored forbade a complete image. And the existing technology was too rudimentary for the time being to fill in the gaps. Howland's question, it appeared, like the mapping of the earth, might be a multigenerational effort.

"Them Thar Hills"

Even if Cobb and Lennox failed to find a clear, succinct answer to Howland's question, something special was happening in Boston. In 1930, Cobb, now 44 years old, was appointed Director of the newly formed neurological unit at Boston City Hospital. Under his Directorship, a powerhouse team of researchers, all united by an intense interest in epilepsy, fortuitously fell into place. Lennox followed Cobb to Boston City Hospital and they were soon joined by a Harvard trained neurosurgeon named Tracy Putnam and a John's Hopkins trained neurologist, Houston Merritt.

Putnam and Merritt met while in the throes of a neurological internship at the hospital and they experienced a powerful connection, forming a deep and enduring friendship. Both were described as "brilliant" and capable of having "unusual insights."

Putman had more than a professional interest in epilepsy because two of his relatives – one a cousin whom he regarded as a sister – suffered from the affliction. Their talent, passion and intellect did not go unnoticed by Cobb, he actively recruited them into the research effort. Together the group formed a tempest of creativity. What happened at Boston City Hospital was a rare alignment of the stars, a group of personalities that collectively elevated their work far beyond any single individual's ability. An uninhibited atmosphere of infectious enthusiasm encouraged bold ideas. A writer described the unit: "its roster establishes the unit among the greatest institutions ever of its kind."

But the timing couldn't have been worse. The fragile realization of the extraordinary research team was almost shattered in its infancy. When the great depression struck in 1930, it crushed research programs across the country. For Cobb and Lennox, when Howland's cash ran out, Harvard rushed to form an "Epilepsy Commission" so their work wouldn't die on the vine. The program was funded by voluntary donations – which shut off like a spigot in the aftermath of Black Tuesday. At the last second, the Rockefeller institute stepped in – if they hadn't, the history of epilepsy treatment may have had its course altered in incalculable ways.

The group knew the largest obstacle to understanding and improving treatments was a lack of good animal models to study. The current models used chemicals to induce seizures – a clumsy and inconsistent method that gave sometimes wildly different results. The newly developed electroencephalographic (EEG) instrument was able to record electrical discharge from patient's brains. When strapped to an epileptic patient's head, through a frantic amplification of squiggles on paper, the machine revealed a tornado of excessive electrical discharge.

No one knew why the storm occurred, where it came from, or what caused it to disappear, but the new machine identified what a seizure was: electrical impulses firing without purpose – an overload of signal pulsating through the brain. Putnam reasoned that if a seizure was an electrical discharge then maybe he could trigger a seizure in animals by the same route: by administering an electric shock. The group seized Putnam's insight. Using parts from an electric motor taken from a salvaged WWI German airplane, they assembled a makeshift machine that would meter out a trigger – a measured electric shock.

After some deliberation, Putman and Merritt decided to test their new machine on cats. The idea was simple: test the cats to see how much of a pulse caused them to have a seizure, then, give the same cats the drug to be tested, wait two hours, and repeat the test. If the cats required more of a shock to trigger a seizure while on the drug, then it was logical to assume the drug was anti-convulsive. Testing known drugs confirmed their logic. When the cats were given bromide it took 50% more current to generate a seizure than before; when given phenobarbital, it took three to four times more current than before. Their model was consistent and reproducible.

The group then made a vital observation. Ever since the discovery of bromides it had always been assumed it was the hypnotic or sedative effect of drugs that muted convulsions – the two properties were inseparable. The new experimental system allowed them to test that assumption. When Putman and Merritt drugged the cats with bromide and phenobarbital to the exact same sedative-state – to the point that prevented the cats from walking – and then used their apparatus to test the seizure threshold – phenobarbital was still much better. This teased out a critical detail. It implied that the sedative property and the

245

anti-convulsive property were not chained together, they could be separated.

They now realized it wasn't necessarily the sedative property of the drugs that made them work. This discovery unshackled the search for new anti-seizure drugs; effectively it removed a massive barrier that had inhibited anti-seizure drug development for about seventy years. The narrow canyon researchers were searching in was suddenly expanded into an open field.

Putnam and Merritt realized the opportunity and began to use their animal model to test new drugs. As modest as it seems on the surface, the experimental system was revolutionary. This was one of the first scaled-up uses of animals to test drugs that might prove useful in humans, a process now called *translational medicine*. Given that phenobarbital was the best drug available, Putnam made a short leap of logic; he would test derivatives of phenobarbital –compounds that were chemically similar.

Their animal model, and method of screening compounds, was Henry Ford's newly developed assembly-line recapitulated into the industry of drug discovery – a quantum leap in productivity. Before the process of drug discovery was mostly accidental, now it was *purposeful*. The system vastly streamlined the probability for successfully finding new drugs because it allowed for screening *en masse* – they would be able to churn through chemicals with untold speed and precision.

Putnam began to search. He combed through the Eastman Chemical company catalog looking for compounds that were structurally just a shade away from phenobarbital. At the same time, he was calling pharmaceutical companies, asking if they had anything that resembled phenobarbital. Specifically, because they had shown the hypnotic quality of anti-seizure drugs was not essential, he requested "compounds that were thought to be hypnotic but had not proven to be." Only one returned Putnam's call, Author Dox, a chemist at Parke-Davis.

At the end of April a package arrived at Boston City Hospital from Dox with Putnam's name on it. Inside, were 7 analogs of phenobarbital and a dozen other compounds that fit Putnam's description. Dox warned Putnam of the futility of what he was trying to accomplish. He told him his search was "a waste of time, because the compounds had already been thoroughly tested and

246

were inactive." But Dox had only tested the compounds for the sedative effect, assuming, like everyone, that was enough to rule them out as anticonvulsive drugs. He was unaware that the Boston group had reason to believe otherwise.

One of the phenobarbital derivatives, called phenytoin, had been sitting on the shelf at Parke-Davis for decades. The company had purchased the compound from a German organic chemist in 1908 hoping it had sedative properties. But when the compound was found to be only mildly sedative it was placed on the shelf in a store room and forgotten. The overlooked compound was first on the list for Putnam and Merritt to test.

They knew it had failed as a sleeping pill, and so had less of a sedative effect than current drugs. When they gave the drug to the cats it was clear they weren't overly impaired; Dox was right, it was only mildly sedative. But when they tested the cat's seizure threshold it left them in astonishment. The drug raised the threshold far beyond the other known drugs, *without heavily sedating them*. This was exactly what they were looking for, the holy grail of epilepsy treatment, a drug that was less sedative yet powerfully anticonvulsive.

The early 1930's were a much different time. Regulators didn't require preclinical safety testing for new drugs (the Food, Drug, and Cosmetic Act was signed in 1938). Nevertheless, just to be sure, Putnam and Merritt handed the drug over to a toxicologist at Harvard, and one at Parke-Davis. Both found phenytoin could be given to cats, dogs, and rats at very high single and repeated doses without immediate toxic effects. This was enough to clear the path and they started treating patients in May.

By the summer of 1938 they had treated 200 adult and pediatric patients with phenytoin, now branded Dilantin, and presented their results at an AMA meeting in San Francisco. The results were remarkable. According to Putnam and Merritt, Dilantin was able to eliminate, or greatly reduce the seizures in 85% of the patients tested. Minor toxic symptoms were reported in 15% of the patients and "more serious toxic reactions" were reported in 5%. Six days later, Parke-Davis added Dilantin to its list of marketed products.

The rest is history. The popularity of the drug grew quickly. By 1940 it was hailed as ushering in a new epoch in the treatment of epilepsy. One doctor called it, "the most remarkable and important chemotherapeutic agent in the convulsive disorders since 1912..." Truly a new era had taken hold for epileptic patients. Across the country, doctors began prescribing Dilantin as a first line treatment for their patients.

The discovery of Dilantin did something else: it aroused and unbridled the capitalistic instinct of pharmaceutical companies. They paid close attention to the discovery of Dilantin. Perhaps even more important than the discovery of Dilantin itself, was the permanent enshrinement of the methodology established by Putnam and Merritt. The significance of Putnam and Merritt's animal model was not lost on big-pharma. The companies quickly established their own in-house large scale drug screening programs. Putnam and Merritt themselves screened over 700 compounds for anti-convulsive activity between 1937 and 1945. The massively scaled-up efforts produced results. Over the next two decades, a dozen new anticonvulsants hit the shelves at the pharmacy.

As quickly as the new era of anticonvulsive drugs was ushered in, the ketogenic diet was ushered out. Dilantin was viewed as modern medicine at its best. It was a symbol of progress, mankind's continuous vector of medical advancement. With the advent of seizure control for many patients in the form of a pill, the onerous diet was soon regarded as "rigid and expensive", and began a sharp decent from favor. A pill was so much easier. A pill took a doctor seconds to scribble its prescription.

The diet took the time and effort of many individuals; the doctor, a dietitian, nurses, and the families. With a pill, everyone was *released*. They no longer had to plan every shopping list and meal. The kids and families could live normal lives. They no longer were cast as outsiders. They could enjoy the same food everybody else was having. They could now have birthday cake, pancakes with syrup, and dessert alongside their friends and family – they didn't have to watch from the sidelines.

History is full of research that drifts off like an unfinished conversation. Alongside the ketogenic diet, Howland's original question faded from relevance. It was a strange query from a by-gone era. How fasting, or the ketogenic diet worked to stop seizures no longer mattered to the vast majority of researchers. But not everyone felt that way. It faded from view with a

248

smattering of unheard protest. At the Mayo clinic, Peterman, found Dilantin "disappointing" compared to the ketogenic diet. Ironically, years later, speaking to a group of resident physicians at the NIH (National Institute of Health, Washington D.C.), Dr. Merritt was rumored to tell the young doctors that his discovery of phenytoin was a major setback to the understanding of epilepsy.

He felt the line of research started by Howland's original question of why fasting worked, and then morphing to the ketogenic diet, was a thread that could have ultimately led to a deeper understanding into the mechanisms of epilepsy. In 1960, almost 40 years after he was recruited to work on Howland's question, Lennox looked back nostalgically, "Though interest in fasting (or the ketogenic diet) as a treatment has almost vanished, doubtless much scientific gold remains in them thar hills".

By 1990, the ketogenic diet was all but completely forgotten. It was a strange, antiquated side-note that most physicians felt belonged in a history book, not a modern textbook. The diet was labeled "rigid, unpalatable, and constraining on daily life." Johns Hopkins, one of the original hospitals to help develop and utilize the diet in the 20's and 30's, barely managed to preserve a single prescribing physician – Dr. John Freeman, and his dietitian, Millicent Kelly, a seventy-two year old that had been administering the diet for forty years. There was vanishingly little demand for their services.

Kelly taught the ketogenic diet to the families of less than 10 children a year. To the doctors around the country, Freeman and Kelly might as well have been a museum exhibit.

Kelly scribbled in an old notepad, calculating ratios and jotting down recipes for the families. "Together, we were the keepers of the flame," Freeman later wrote. Besides Kelly, so few dietitians were trained in the nuances of the diet that when it was used, it was administered sloppily, and the children often had bad outcomes.

The lessons of the past, that it took precise calculations to achieve the best seizure control, were all but lost. The bad results were folded into the perception that the diet was old, outdated, and not as effective as the current drugs. The widespread opinion was that the diet "did not work and was difficult to tolerate" and its use was "no longer justified." Across the country, its use became almost nonexistent.

"Wait a Minute, This Didn't Have to Happen"

As the Abrahamses flew to Baltimore for the last remaining chance to treat Charlie's unremitting seizures, their thoughts cartwheeled between sadness, desperation, and the last sliver of hope. Most likely they were experiencing the same emotions as the Howlands as they rode the train toward Battle Creek eighty years earlier. As he traversed the American landscape, Abrahams was entirely unaware of the rich history surrounding the ketogenic diet as a treatment for epilepsy. That it was once the standard-of-care for epilepsy would have shocked and bewildered him even more so.

For Abrahams, and most doctors and patients across the country, the ketogenic diet was *dead* – reduced to the equivalent of an herbalist working out of a strip mall.

When they arrived at Johns Hopkins they met with Dr. Freeman and his dietitian, Millicent Kelly. The pair seemed perfectly matched. Dr. Freeman was the maverick. "He was larger than life; fearless; he knew he was considered an outlier by a lot of his colleagues, but in a way I think that intrigued him." Millicent was the soft side – comforting, Grandmother-like mannerisms that were amplified to almost cartoonish levels. With a charming and soothing voice that seemed to round the edges of every word, she explained the diet to Abrahams. With no time to spare, they began the diet with a jump start, they fasted Charlie the rest of the day and into the next.

By the next day, when Abrahams held his son he could already tell a difference; he just felt "less intense", like something had been turned down. By the next day, forty-eight hours later, something remarkable happened: his son stopped having seizures. *Completely*. The Abrahamses returned home brimming with optimism and hope. Days passed, and then weeks, and the seizures remained at bay.

The diet had an incredibly powerful impact. It had done what of drugs and surgery were unable to do; it had brought his son back from the abyss. Charlie began to thrive. His mental capacity and energy returned. The house, once filled with tears, was now filled with joy.

The story of the Abrahamses would have ended there – they would have been just one of the ten or so that Dr. Freeman and Millicent quietly helped every year. But like Howland before him, the experience aroused something deep. Medicine had failed them. Things begin to stir in Abrahams when he returned to his normal life. Something just didn't sit well. "All of a sudden my eyes opened up in the middle of the night, and I said 'wait a minute, this didn't have to happen.' Ninety percent of these seizures didn't have to occur.

Waking up around the clock, and pouring drugs down his throat, didn't have to occur." Abrahams' epiphany morphed into puzzlement and anger. What motivated him the most is that he was in a position to prevent this from happening to others.

Where Howland had the money of a wealthy corporate lawyer, Abrahams had something even better – perhaps the best resource in the world for taking up a cause: Hollywood. Abrahams had produced blockbuster hits like Airplane, Naked Gun, and Hot Shots. If it was simply a lack of information, he could change that. So he and his wife Nancy started the now famous Charlie Foundation dedicated to disseminating information about the ketogenic diet so Charlie's story would not be repeated. On October 26th, 1994, the NBC news program Dateline brought Charlie's story into millions of living rooms across the country.

At the end of the show viewers were given a number to call. Families that called were sent a video from the Charlie Foundation titled *An Introduction to the Ketogenic Diet*. The foundation also mailed the same tape to neurologists throughout the country. Shortly after, neurologists were mailed another video titled *The Ketogenic Diet: Doctors Version*. It was a well-orchestrated plan and its impact was enormous. Abrahams also had the Charlie foundation ready to fund a seven-center trial designed to measure the impact of the ketogenic diet once and for all. A trial would serve to demonstrate the efficacy of the forgotten diet for both patients and doctors.

It was timed perfectly. Shortly before the Dateline special the Charlie Foundation quietly had doctors, dietitians, nurses, and families with an epileptic child come to Johns Hopkins and receive intensive training on the use of the proven Johns Hopkins ketogenic diet protocol. The doctors and their staffs were then ready and waiting for the anticipated surge of new patients coming from media blitz that began with the prime-time Dateline special. As expected, the kids came from all corners of the country, desperate to try the new diet. Four years later Freeman published the results from 150 kids that entered the trial. The patient group enrolled in the trial was a tough lot.

As a group, they averaged 410 seizures per month and had already failed to improve after trying an average of 6.2 medications. Nevertheless, the outcome was dramatic. Of the 55% still on the diet after a year, 27% were close to seizure free, 23% were significantly improved, and the remaining 5% had a less than 50% reduction of seizures. Three to six years later, 27% of these same children had few to no seizures and most were off of the diet and on fewer to no medication.

To further raise public awareness, a year before the data from the trial was published, Abrahams released an ABC television movie titled *First Do No Harm* starring his good friend Meryl Streep. It was the dramatic portrayal of a Midwestern family's struggle to find the ketogenic diet for their child with severe and unresponsive epilepsy. Eight million viewers watched the movie the night it was aired.

In truth, the Charlie Foundation's clinical trial just confirmed the results of the thirteen other studies that had been performed since Wilder first purposed the diet as a treatment in 1921. The only difference this time, because of Jim Abrahams' elegantly choreographed media campaign, people were paying attention. The study was presented at the annual American Epilepsy Society in 1996. Before the study was presented, the ketogenic diet was almost never mentioned at the annual gathering. But this time, combined with the media firestorm, it precipitated an avalanche of research the following year, and only grew in the years after that. The ketogenic diet had been resurrected – as quickly as it had fallen, because of the discovery of Dilantin, it had been revived by a passionate family and their sick child.

————

Seven minutes and fifty-five seconds into the Dateline special featuring Charlie's story, Charlie's doctor, Donald Shields, said something important. The reporter asked Dr. Shields: "You had some knowledge this diet was probably working back at Johns Hopkins (Dr. Shields and Dr. Freeman were actually good friends), yet you dissuaded the Abrahams from attempting it, how come?" Dr. Shields paused, looked at the ceiling, and said, "Well, because I don't think we had exhausted all of the medical approaches yet. There were actually other medications we hadn't tried yet." Drawing a distinction between so called "medical approaches" and the ketogenic diet reveals volumes of the way many doctors view the dietary protocol – something existing outside of the realm of real medicine – something strange, nonconventional, and alternative. Why else would the diet have faded into complete obscurity in the first place?

Even today the diet is rarely used as a first line treatment. It is still something held in reserve. Epilepsy is almost always treated first with drugs. Medication will make half of the patient's seizure free for an extended period of time. But if a patient doesn't respond to the first drug the odds rapidly diminish. In these cases a second drug will only make an additional 14% seizure free.

If that drug fails then the likelihood of seizure control using drugs falls to about 1 to 2 percent. Remarkably, even with the most recent anti-seizure drugs, these ratios have remained essentially the same throughout the century– as if some fundamental barrier cannot be breached by drugs alone. So that leaves more than 30% of epileptic patients without seizure control even with the latest, and best medications.

Before Abrahams pulled the diet from obscurity, these patients had nowhere to turn. Today, this is where the ketogenic diet is typically used – as an option of last resort. For the over 30% of patients with uncontrolled seizures after failing drug therapy the ketogenic diet is a godsend. If maintained properly, it renders half of this desperate group either completely or extremely close to seizure free. These incredible results have been shown consistently in study after study throughout the 20th century. In addition, most kids who use the diet can transition back to a normal western diet after two years, never need drugs again, and remain seizure free.

After combing through the statistics an inevitable question arises: why is the diet only held as an option of last resort? One can't help but wonder: which is better as a first-line treatment, drugs, or the ketogenic diet? To be sure, the comparisons, from trials alone, are not apples to apples. A direct head to head comparison has never been done. The answer to this question remains unknown.

However, there is a very important difference between the studies of anti-seizure drugs and the ketogenic diet: all of the modern studies of the ketogenic diet use a patient population that has failed drug treatment. The dietary trials have a built-in bias from the starting line. The tests done on the ketogenic diet are enrolled with the hardest cases – patients with gritty, embedded seizures that refuse to be blunted by the best medications available.

"You've already peeled off the easiest cases. It's like running a one-hundred yard dash with a weight chained to your leg," said Dr. James Wheless, a pediatric neurologist, and a recognized expert on the use of the ketogenic diet. Even in the face of such difficult odds, the ketogenic diet shows incredible results.

Of course, any comparison of diet verses drugs must also include side effects. Even modern drugs aren't completely benign. When Charlie was saturated in anti-seizure drugs Abrahams described him as a "zombie who lived in his car seat." Although technology has continued to separate the sedative effect and the anti-seizure effect, it is not perfect. Drugs often leave patients lethargic, dizzy, and with double vision. Rashes appear, weight gain, abnormal liver function, kidney stones, and constipation.

The biggest difference between anti-seizure medication and the ketogenic diet occurs in the brain. Indeed, the brain is ground zero in the debate of diet versus drugs. The side effects that occur from medication are not there in the diet, in fact, the opposite occurs. Doctors today notice the same mental effects as the original pioneers of the diet back at the beginning of the 20th century: increased alertness, improved behavior, reduced anxiety and depression. How the patient experiences life is markedly different between drugs and the diet – a variable that defies quantification.

The strict form of the diet is not without some issues. Side effects do occur, but they are very minor, including changes in lipid profiles, kidney stones, constipation, and a subtle slowing of growth. However, improvements in the diet formulation, macronutrient sources, supplements, and interventions have greatly diminished lipid abnormalities, constipation and kidney stones.

A 2010 study at Johns Hopkins followed the outcomes of children treated with the ketogenic diet from 1993 to 2008 and found almost no long-term adverse effects. The only obvious effect was growth. Height was found to be reduced by 5 cm from the *expected* average.

All other laboratory values were normal. Most importantly, the study found the subjects had continued to either maintain, or improve on seizure control, even into adulthood. Most of the families had few regrets and would recommend the diet to others. All added up – results combined with side-effects – many experts in the field give a nod to the ketogenic diet when directly compared to drugs. They feel the diet is often simply the best medical option. "No anticonvulsive drugs have that rate of beneficial effect," wrote Dr. Freeman.

Despite the heroic efforts of Abrahams, his wife Nancy, and the Charlie Foundation, the ketogenic diet is still today underutilized. When an epileptic child enters a neurologist's practice the typical scenario goes like this: the patient is prescribed a first-line drug. As stated above, this works about half of the time. For the half that fail to respond, the neurologist will prescribe another drug.

This time the drug works in about one in seven kids (it doesn't matter which drug is chosen, the statistics remain the same). For the kids that don't respond to the second drug the neurologist will now almost always try a third. The chance the third drug will work now falls to one percent. This leaves over one in three kids that come back to the neurologist office in a desperate situation, after having failed three drugs. The neurologist now has a decision to make. According to a 2008 special report issued by a consortium of 26 world-recognized experts using the ketogenic diet from nine countries, this is precisely where the diet should be prescribed, after the failure of two to three drugs.

At this point the data begs to be heard: the ketogenic diet will make over half of this desperate group of kids either entirely, or very close to seizure free – the other half simply can't or won't maintain the diet for a variety of reasons – either they find the diet isn't working, or it's too hard to maintain. Prescribing a fourth drug has a vanishingly small chance of working. Yet, strangely, in many cases, the neurologist will keep going; writing script after script for more and more drugs – many never suggesting the diet – the same dreadful place Charlie and his family found themselves.

When I asked Jim if Charlie's "story" still happens today, he responded in a sober tone: "Sadly, Yes. And in many ways its worse; the reason is because there are more drugs. The physicians frequently say, 'well there is another drug, let's try that instead.' From what we see, from those who contact us, I don't know the exact statics, but rarely is the diet prescribed after the failure of two or three medications." Why the diet continues to be marginalized is a poignant question. "It's a culture shift," said Dr. Wheless. "The mindset today is to take a pill and be done. If the diet was in pill form it would be the best treatment available."

It raises an important question. Are we as a culture, both patients and physicians, willing to marginalize an incredibly effective therapy at the expense of some convenience? The question is especially relevant considering the price paid is so incredibly high. "One of the things that pisses me off the most is that the whole degree of difficulty thing; it's not a medical question," said Abrahams.

"When you're holding your kid while he has hundreds of seizures a day, and then you find out doctors aren't giving you all the information...because they think, 'it's too difficult' – where in medical school did they teach a course on what's considered too difficult for the parents of a critically ill child."

To get this right is not trivial. Epilepsy affects 65 million people across the globe – almost one percent of the world's population. The most updated statistic released by the CDC claim 1 in 26 people will develop epilepsy at some point in their life. Despite extensive testing, over half of all cases are idiopathic, meaning no reason for the illness can be found. It mostly affects children, but can also affect adults – the chances increasing with age. It is a terrifying disease because there are so many unknowns.

Still today, after centuries of investigation, researchers cannot tell you exactly what a seizure is, where it comes from, or why it stops. Words crop up like "multifactorial", and "network effect"; which, although true, are really a way of saying "we don't know exactly" – a bucket to throw very difficult problems in. Epilepsy erodes at the edges of life, interrupting, stealing, and isolating its victims. It is not passive. Over time, if severe enough, epilepsy won't allow the brain to develop correctly. It is a tremendous burden for societies across the globe. And to let an extraordinary therapy remain under prescribed because of an undefined apathy is tragic and deserves an explanation.

Near the end of the Dateline special featuring Charlies story, the reporter asked Dr. Shields a final question: "Dr. Freeman tells us that fifty to seventy percent of the patients that come through his doors and get put on the ketogenic diet have success. Can you think of any drugs, in these hard cases, that have fifty to seventy percent success rates?" Dr. Shield's again looked to the ceiling before answering, "Probably not anything that comes up to that level." After some reflection, Dr. Shields backpedaled, and came up with a possible explanation for this astonishing situation – a reason why the diet is so often ignored. "There is no big drug company behind the ketogenic diet.

And there will never be unless somebody starts marketing sausage and eggs with cream sauce on it as a drug." Abrahams agrees with Dr. Shield's assessment about why the diet remains in the shadows, "It's not in the form of a pill, it can't be administered with a scalpel, and the only people who profit from the ketogenic diet are the patients," said Abrahams.

At the front-line of the Charlie Foundation's efforts is their head nutritionist Beth Zupec-Kania. Over her 24 years with the Charlie Foundation Beth has trained dietitians in 10 countries and treated thousands of epileptic patients around the world. Perhaps more than anyone, she has witnessed the power of the ketogenic diet to treat epilepsy first hand. Typically, when she sees a patient they are on at least two anti-seizure drugs, have failed many more, are sick, frustrated, and exhausted.

The patients that finally turn to the diet do so for more than one reason, said Zupec-Kania, "Their seizures continue unabated, or they are experiencing such severe side-effects that they are essentially nonfunctional, or both. Sadly, it's *usually both*." Most are left simmering in a state of pronounced lethargy because of the drugs.

Some drugs are worse than others. "The worst drug is Topamax", said Zupec-Kania. "The nickname that the doctors
258

call it behind the backs of patients is 'Dope-a-max' because it makes you feel so dopey. The patients can't think of words that they used to know." With the diet, she says that parents often notice a marked mental improvement once the child achieves ketosis. And this improvement occurs *while the patients are on the same amount of drugs.* Neurologists typically won't start reducing the drugs until the patient has maintained the diet for at least a month; after it's clear they are tolerating it well. The difference is striking.

"All of a sudden the kid is paying attention, or stringing words together, kind of coming out of a fog," said Zupec-Kania. "Jim has a video of this mom describing her six year old son: 'he got up, he went to the bathroom, he cleaned up, and he came back to bed, and he hadn't done that in the past year.' The moment he went into ketosis he got his life back."

Zupec-Kania said the short term side effects from the diet are preventable and researchers have yet to find any long term side effects. In fact, she has a different take. "I think these patients are healthier because of what they are not eating. Having worked with thousands of people, many of them will continue leaving processed foods and sugar out of their diets and are healthier in the long run," she says. Through her quarter century of experience she has also made another striking observation.

The ridged boundaries of the diet, the 4 to 1 ratio that has been the 'gold standard' for patients, may not be as vital to achieving seizure control as once thought. "Lots of patients probably don't need the full blown ketogenic diet to get better; we could probably use something far more liberal and have the same effect. And I'm not even talking about the Modified Atkins Diet (which is used mainly for adolescents and adults with epilepsy),

I'm talking about a paleo-type diet. I spoke to a mom last night who said her son just started having seizures out of the blue and after her nutritionist eliminated wheat and sugar from his diet his seizures stopped immediately. I would love to spare some people of the difficulty of the rigid form of the diet if it's not needed. And now we're finding just a low glycemic index diet can work in some cases. There is a whole spectrum of people and a whole spectrum of diets to meet their needs.

Dr. Jung Rho, of the University of Calgary is on the forefront of the current effort to answer Howland's original question. For Rho, the question remains as haunting today as it did in 1921. Rho is nearing the end of a $2 million dollar, five year grant from the NIH to find the mechanism behind the ketogenic diet's action on epilepsy. And as with those that came before him – Cobb, Lennox, Gamble, and Dr. Howland –the answer, wrote Rho, "remains elusive". Rho's estimation of the diet's effect is essentially the same as Lennox's *"stones forming a mosaic"* description almost a century ago: "At present, there are many hypotheses regarding KD (ketogenic diet) action, and while each is uniquely compelling, it is becoming more apparent that the KD likely works through multiple mechanisms," wrote Rho.

It's not surprising Rho and others have yet to pin down the diet's exact mechanism-of-action, given the nature of the human brain; an organ with 125 trillion neural synapses just in the cerebral cortex alone, a number roughly equal to the number of stars in 1,500 Milky Way galaxies.

That level of staggering complexity, combined with the fact the pathophysiological mechanism behind seizures is still largely unknown, appears to have rendered Howland's question *still* out of our technological reach. Perhaps the most important realization from Rho's research is a deeper understanding of the nature of epilepsy: "The scientific literature involving the KD strongly supports the notion that epilepsy may indeed in part represent a "metabolic disease", and that this concept could serve as a novel framework for the development of more effective anti-seizure drugs," wrote Rho in July of 2015.

"The Genie is Out of the Bottle"

Even though, within the largely incentive driven arena of medicine, the ketogenic diet is still clearly under-prescribed today as a therapy for epilepsy, Jim Abrahams single-handedly managed to thrust the forgotten therapy back into the public and scientific consciousness. Before his Hollywood fueled campaign, the diet lie dormant – an artifact – after, researchers were once again stirred by the curious power of the ketogenic diet. Jim unknowingly resurrected a query from a by-gone era. To any curious biochemist, it is *still* astonishing in its own right that a simple shift in macromolecular consumption could have such a profound effect on brain chemistry.

By the late 1990's, researchers turned their attention and laboratory space over to the ketogenic diet with revolutionary zeal. The number of researcher papers containing the phrase "ketogenic diet" exploded – from only two-hundred and twenty-five before the year 2000, to one-thousand four-hundred in the fifteen years after the year 2000. The earlier articles published were almost exclusively about the role of the diet in epilepsy, but around the turn of the century researchers had begun to nudge at the margins of the diet, exploring its possible role beyond epilepsy. Researchers, for the first time, began asking other questions of the diet: could it be used to treat or prevent other diseases?

First it was cancer in 1995. It was a tiny study – only two little girls with brain cancer – but the results hinted at a potent impact and precipitated an avalanche of research into ketosis and cancer. As biochemists uncovered the unique mechanistic-details of ketosis it opened new possibilities. One paper, in 2003, by NIH scientist Richard Veech and George Cahill, was a siren call.

Specifically, it suggested the ketogenic diet, or ketone bodies by themselves, had the potential to affect a wide swath of pathologic conditions precipitated by insulin resistance and dysfunctional mitochondrial metabolism – fundamental processes that can lead to a constellation of problems. "What are the potential uses of beta-hydroxybutyrate in addition to pediatric epilepsy?" asked Veech, "Theoretically, any condition wherein oxygen supply to cells may be limited is an avenue for investigation. The list would encompass almost every disease state." The paper was a foot in the door, behind which was an open-ended spectrum of possibility.

Other researchers took notice. Studies on physical performance, Alzheimer's, and depression began in 2004. Parkinson's disease, traumatic brain injury, type 2 diabetes, Lafora body disease, polycystic ovary syndrome (PCOS), and metabolic syndrome in 2005, amyotrophic lateral sclerosis (ALS or Lou Gehrig's disease) in 2006, nonalcoholic fatty liver disease in 2007.

Incredibly, perhaps counterintuitively, the ketogenic diet showed promise to "modify" the course of one disease after the next. The strangely vast spectrum of diseases the diet appeared to attenuate caught many researchers off guard. Clearly, the diet was able to shift metabolism and genetic expression at some base level that prevented, rejuvenated, and protected cells, tissues, and organs (notably the brain) from the accumulation of disease causing damage. Like epilepsy, in most cases the exact influence ketones were having on the variety of diseases remained elusive. Howland's question became vastly expanded.

The Charlie Foundation became a conduit for the ketogenic diet's sudden expansion in interest. The calls, once dominated by the pleas of epileptic patients, made an abrupt shift to other diseases. Now, around the turn of the century, when the phone rang, or an email came it, it was most likely a cancer patient, or someone with Alzheimer's, or Parkinson's, or other more obscure problems. The Foundation decided to evolve, and allowed itself to be led be the science. They changed their name from The *Charlie Foundation for pediatric epilepsy* to The *Charlie Foundation for ketogenic therapies.*

Suddenly Zupec-Kania found herself teaching the diet to a vastly expanded group of health professionals. "We get more calls from cancer patients than epileptics now," she said. Zupec-Kania has noticed the utility of the diet continues to heave and undulate, covering additional ailments; its circle of effectiveness, surprisingly, continues to expand. "I'm getting more and more calls from people with migraines which 16% of Americans suffer from. We've found out the diet is super effective for migraines. And surprisingly, the other one is hot flashes from menopause.

The ketogenic diet, even a liberal ketogenic diet, cures hot flashes."

For most of history epilepsy was viewed as a supernatural possession. Even today, vestiges of a mystical dimension linger. We know the disease is biological in origin, but it remains an enigma, it transcends our ability to succinctly explain it. That a subtle shift in energy metabolism is able to exorcise epileptic fits evokes imagery of preternatural healing; a biological force beyond our understanding. Incredibly, the discovery that the beneficial transition to ketone metabolism extends far past epilepsy, into unimaginable arenas of disease, only carries this image further – as evocative as it is astonishing.

The literature reflects this feeling; words like "magical, superfuel, jet-fuel, and magic bullet," slip from the pens of typically skeptical, objective and clinical scientists. The turn of the century marked the transition. The door is now open to a new era of medicine that, refreshingly, might have more to do with prevention than the never-ending cat and mouse game of diagnosing and treating disease after they have become intractably embedded – a game that is almost by definition, impossible to win. But it even goes beyond prevention.

Ketone research has seduced us into imagining it might be possible to lift ourselves onto even higher planes of health and vitality. A bold new era of medicine beckons. Never have we asked if our health can be elevated, optimized, and extended with such vast technological resources at our fingertips.

The hybrid nature of human metabolism to utilize ketones as an energy source was not fully appreciated until the 1960's. And even then it was typically confused with diabetic ketoacidosis – a pathological condition that has nothing to do with fasting or nutritional ketosis in general. Nevertheless the two were lumped together and the true disease modifying potential of nutritional ketosis was not fully appreciated until around the turn of the century.

We now know, the shift to ketone metabolism goes far beyond the swapping of one fuel for another. Hidden just below the surface we've uncovered a new layer of complexity: we now know ketones are absolutely profound in their impact to human physiology. Critically, they act as signaling molecules and carry deeply conserved messages to our DNA – messages that vastly impact our overall health.

Ketones change the architecture of our DNA, rearranging the way it is expressed, turning on the same rejuvenating pathways stimulated by caloric restriction or periodic fasting. Ketones appear to powerfully reduce inflammatory pathways – the smoldering process that is blamed for a vast spectrum of problems, even a reduction of overall lifespan. There is a growing consensus that most of the so called modern disease of civilization – obesity, type 2 diabetes, and Alzheimer's (now called type 3 diabetes), cancer and many others – all ripple outward from a central core of metabolic dysfunction.

These modern diseases, once considered pathologically distinct, converge to the same central place – a place that ketone metabolism concentrates its profoundly rejuvenating and repairing capacity. As Dr. Veech has said, "Ketosis is a normal physiological state. I would argue it is the normal state of man. It's not normal to have a McDonald's and a Delicatessen on every corner. It's normal to starve." Perhaps many of our modern ailments are a result of stepping too far from our natural state of existence.

It's easy to recognize the societal resistance to any rigid dietary adjustment and the search is underway to find shortcuts. "The 20th century was about understanding the ketogenic diet," said Dr. Wheless. "The 21st century is going to be about trying to capture its incredible benefits in a pill."

Science is a building that is constantly under construction. The progress we are making today rises from a foundation built by others. In addition to all those mentioned in the article, the work of Drs. Richard Veech, Sami Hashim and Henri Brunengraber has laid the concrete that we in this field all work and build. These metabolic gurus were responsible for opening the blinds and illuminating the therapeutic potential of exogenous ketone supplementation.

Standing on the shoulders of these giants, our laboratory at University of South Florida has been studying the effects of ketone supplementation on numerous disease states, physical performance and resilience against extreme environments. Could these small molecules – once thought to be metabolic waste – hold the potential to treat and prevent a constellation of

264

metabolic related illness? Do they capture the time honored benefits of caloric restriction or intermittent fasting? Can they enhance our health, vitality and longevity – allowing the baby boomers, a generation that refuses to *"go gently into that good night"*, to extract more from life for longer?

The initial results look promising.the data emerging rapidly from studies on nutritional ketosis are compelling and have far reaching implications. Perhaps Jim Abrahams said it best: "The genie is out of the bottle."

Chapter 7 - Bonus Text: What is the RockSolid Diet?

aka
How to improve your Omega 6 to Omega 3 ratio – by avoiding seed oils [Nov 2022}

[I include this text here because I think that too much Omega 6 fatty acids are the main reason, that your mitochondria get broken in the first place. Because of damaged Cardiolipin. See Tucker Goodrich, Chris Knobbe and Paul Saladino on more information on this. It is not included because Prof. Seyfried said so, it is just my own idea.]

IMPORTANT: This is a revised transcript of the video I made, it was published on my YouTube Channel "The RockSolidDiet".
It has way more pictures than displayed here in it, also there are lot of elaborate *Star Wars* effects and clips in it. So you can just watch the video here, it is about 1 our long and divided in 6 chapters:

https://youtu.be/SUoqWbEntKc

BUT PLEASE: To help me with the YouTube algorithm, **please watch the video in its FULL LENGTH.** If it's really too long, you don't have to be in front of the screen to make it count :-p Or just watch in separate sessions.
Maybe also subscribe, like and leave comment... as a reward for this Bonus Text. Thanks a lot!
Also: If you wanna give this text to friends and family, especially the ones over 40 that have a family history of a DOC, then you can buy the eBook for just 4,90 Dollars on Amazon. Thanks for your support!
Title: *"The RockSolid Diet: Prevent and heal cancer, heart disease, diabetes and obesity – By avoiding toxic Omega 6 fats in vegetable & seed oils (Linoleic Acid)"*
Okay, here you go: How can you prevent the diseases of civilisation, especially cancer? By following the ROCKSOLID DIET. Enjoy!

Introduction and Outline

You want to know what the RockSolid Diet is? Okay! And - you will also learn, how you can use the RockSolid Diet to improve your Omega 6 to 3 ratio. Because the RockSolid Diet is about avoiding the Omega 6s that are in seed oils.

Following the RockSolid Diet will prevent you of getting sick of the so-called "Diseases of civilisation" – like cancer, heart disease, diabetes and obesity.

Let's take a look at the outline:

1) In Chapter 1, you will learn about the Omega 6 to Omega 3 ratio – and why you can never get that ratio right. I will also tell you, what the definition of *RockSolid* exactly is.
2) Chapter 2 is about the real cause of the DOCs, the diseases of civilisation. As an example, we will talk about heart disease and Ancel Keys' Diet-Heart-Hypothesis.
3) In the 3rd chapter, you will learn what food items contribute the most to our Omega 6 consumption and how much our current intake is.
4) Chapter number 4 is about the *Animal Fat Anomaly.*
5) In chapter 5 we will do the math on how much Omega 6 you are actually allowed to eat.
6) And finally, in chapter 6, I will present to you my own, home-made, Omega 6 calculator – and show you how to use it!

Okay, let's get it on!

Chapter 1:
The Omega 6 to Omega 3 Ratio

When it comes to a healthy diet, you likely heard this phrase a thousand times, coming from scientists and experts - what all of those guys want to tell you is:

„Hey buddy! Seems like nutrition science has figured out one thing for sure: If you want to live a healthy and happy life, you should eat less of those nasty Omega 6s - and more of those super awesome Omega 3s!

For the best results, your ratio shouldn't be higher than 2 to 1. Meaning, 2 parts Omega 6s to 1 part Omega 3."

Yeah, that's what the experts say. But: What is our current ratio? I got to tell you, it's really bad! As you can see in this graph here, in 2000, we were already at 16 to 1.

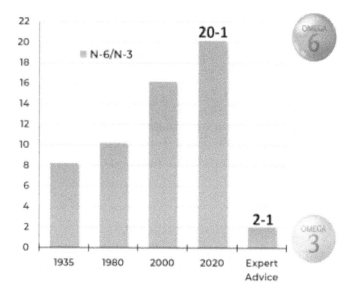

And now, in 2020, we are at 20 to 1! And here, at the very end, that's the ratio that experts recommend: 2 to 1.

But... yeah, what are you going to do with that kind of information? *How* do you get that Omega balance right? Are you going to supplement with fishoil?

Before we go any further, let's quickly take a look at the sources of Omega 3s and 6s in our food supply.

As you may know: Omega 3 fatty acids are predominantly in animal products, especially in fish and seafood, but also in: Meat, organs, dairy and eggs.

These fatty acids are known as EPA and DHA.

They are also labeled as PUFAs: *Poly Unsaturated Fatty Acids.*

Important fact: You can pretty much forget about plant sources of Omega 3, like ALA: ALA has to be converted by our bodies to be usable. Unfortunately, the conversion rate is extremely low, at around 4%.

On the other hand, those "plant Omega 3 sources" contain plenty of Omega 6 – so just forget about them! They only seem healthy, at first glance.

Omega 6s on the other hand are fatty acids, that are predominantly in plant foods.

We eat them normally in the form of grains and seeds, as these are pretty high in fat, and so high in Omega 6s. Examples of direct consumption would be our all-beloved wheat and wheat flour, and pretty much all nuts.

But the way in which we eat the most Omega 6s is quite obvious: We eat them as **oils!** But only since the 19th century, since we humans invented a bunch of technologies to extract those fats and concentrate them. It's a very unnatural process! These oils are all made in factorys and heated up over and over again, which makes them supertoxic

You may call them seed oils, vegetable oils or cooking oils.

Examples are sunflower oil, canola oil or: The famous and infamous soybean oil!

We will also call them "Linoleic Acid" because that's the most abundant Omega 6 fatty acid in them.

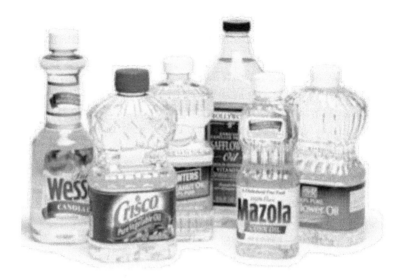

Okay, now that everybody is on the same page, let's get back to our ratio:

The question still is: *How do you get that Omega 6 to Omega 3 balance right?*

Everybody will tell you „Yeah, increase those Omega 3s, man! It's easy: Simply eat more fatty fish! Or supplement with fishoil!"

The Problem is: With our current Omega 6 consumption, you can raise your Omega 3 intake as much as you want – you will never ever get to a 2 to 1 ratio of those fatty acids.

Want proof? Okay!

How much Omega 6 do you think we're eating in a day? What number can you imagine?

Let's see! This graph shows the Omega 6 consumption in the United States from 1909 until 2009.

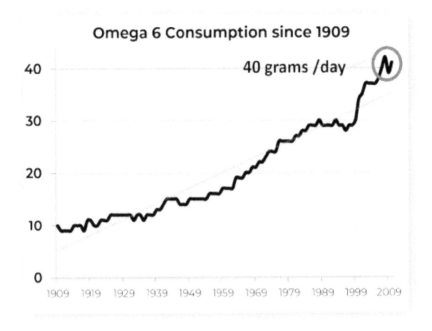

Omega 6 Consumption since 1909

40 grams /day

And, as you can see: In the US, we are currently at **40 grams** of Omega 6 fatty acids per day.

So if you want to get this proper ratio of 2 to 1... and you don't want to change your Omega 6 intake then...

You would have to eat 20 grams of Omega 3 fats. Meaning about 67 fishoil capsules. *Every single day.*

Okay, okay. You don't want to swallow a couple dozen of fishoil capsules? You can, of course, *just eat* 2.5 pounds of salmon a day. Sure, you could do that...

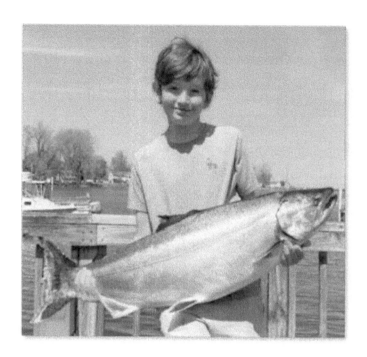

But, come on. Thats a million calories and it would cost you 10,000 dollars a month. It's just a stupid idea overall.

This huge imbalance between Omega 6s and 3s is the reason, that a lot of studies regarding the health benefits of Omega 3 fats didn't get any positive results: Because the few grams of Omega 3s didn't stand a chance against a mountain of Omega 6s.

Now, the very best way to get that ratio right is to simply **eliminate** Omega 6s as much as possible!

And by the way... Omega 6s have turned out to be **extremely unhealthy!** In the last years, a lot of research has come out that proves this.

> *DR. CHRIS KNOBBE:*
> "It is the seed oils that are the primary drivers because they are the biological poisons."
> *DR. PAUL SALADINO:*
> "There is so much good evidence, that polyunsaturated fat is horrible for humans."
> *TUCKER GOODRICH:*

"Seed oils: This thing that turns into a metabolic toxin in your body."

So, it seems that all along, it was not about the RATIO – it was all about the *avoidance* of Omega 6s that was the real health benefit!

Long story short: Omega 6s, also known as seed oils, PUFAS or linoleic acid are poisonous, toxic, and a bunch of other terrible things. So: Just don't eat them!

As I said, a bunch of experts have figured this out. They're saying: "Stop eating seed oils! Avoid them as much as possible!"

But, here's the problem: Nobody ever tells you *how* to really do it. How should you eliminate them? Okay, you switch from cooking with sunflower oil to cooking with coconut oil, alrighty. But then... is that really enough?

This is where the **RockSolid Diet** comes into play! It's all about eliminating Omega 6s.

You probably have asked yourself: What does the RockSolid Diet mean? What is it exactly?

Well, ROCK SOLID stands for

R O C K - Reduction Of Chronik Sickness
through a
S O L I D - Seed Oil Limitation Diet!
You also could say eliminiation diet.

Yeah... obvious, right? It's as easy as that!

The RockSolid Diet is about giving you practical advice and tools on how to reduce Omega 6 fats in real, every day life.

We will tell you

- How much Omega 6 you can eat,
- How you can assess the Omega 6 content of foods and, accordingly,
- What foods to buy and eat!

Well, it's really rather what foods to not eat.
Going back to the unhealthy aspects of these plant fats:
Why specifically should we limit those Omega 6s anyway?

Chapter 2:
The rise and cause of the diseases of civilisation

Everybody has heard of the DOCs, the diseases of civilisation. There are plenty of explanations, why they increased that much since the last 100, 200 years. Because before then, they didn't really exist.

From a nutritional standpoint, it seems quite striking that the inception of Omega 6s **correlates greatly** with all of our current diseases of civilisation.

Let's hear it from Dr. Chris Knobbe. He's going to tell us how these chronic diseases were not really a thing - and how they developed into this big threat that they are today:

DR. CHRIS KNOBBE:
"This is Jones' paper from 2011: What he shows is that in 1900, the top three causes of death were all infectious diseases. It was pneumonia, tuberculosis, GI infections.

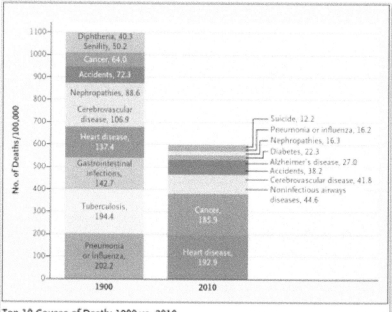

Top 10 Causes of Death: 1900 vs. 2010.

Data are from the Centers for Disease Control and Prevention.

Whereas by 2010, seven of the top ten causes of disease are all chronic diseases: Heart disease, cancer, stroke, Alzheimer's Disease, type 2 diabetes, all that. Let's walk through heart disease over the last 200 years.

From Jones' paper, we know that in the town of Boston in 1811, there were *no heart disease deaths listed.* There was 25 sudden deaths, probably most of those were cardiac valvular.

In the entire 19th century, there's eight worldwide papers - reports essentially - of heart disease. Extraordinarily rare disorder!

1897: Sir William Osler, famed physician of John Hopkins'. He recounts in his previous 21 years of hospital history about six cases of angina. *He had never seen seen a heart attack.*

1900: Jones' paper tells us that 12.5 percent of people died of heart-related disease, but it was virtually all cardiac valvular. There was syphilis, endocarditis, rheumatic fever. It wasn't coronary *artery* disease related, right?

1912: John Herrick publishes the first known case of heart attack in the United States, documented. And documented with autopsy evidence.

In the 1930s, though: Heart disease becomes the leading cause of death - virtually unknown 30 years earlier! In fact, when John Herrick published the paper about the MI, it wasn't even taken seriously for about a decade!

Advance forward to 2010: 32 percent of Americans dying of heart disease, virtually one in three.

Cancer. Boston, 1811: One in 188 people died of cancer. 1900, it's rising, one in 17 in the US. 2010: 31.1 percent of people die of cancer! Right? That's almost, again, one in three.

And what I hear all the time is "Yeah, but we're getting older!" I'm telling you, that does not explain this (...)

So, back to cancer here:

A 62-fold increase in cancer in 200 years!

How about type 2 diabetes? We know, in the 19th century, diabetes of any type was rare and was presumably rare for all of history prior. 1935, it's rising, 0.37 percent. This continues to rise, and we're at 9.4 percent by 2015. This is a 25-fold increase in type 2 diabetes in 80 years!

How about obesity? 19th century: We know that obesity was 1.2 percent in men, age 18 to 80, in Texas and Nebraska prisons. Okay. Look at this: By 1960, we're at 13% obesity. That was a 10-fold increase already! Right? When we thought we were lean.

So this continues to rise and by 2015, we're at 39.8 percent obesity. This is a 33-fold increase in obesity in about 115 years - and we are on target to be at 50 percent of Americans being obese by 2030, that was published in JAMA just a few weeks ago."

In this graph, I summarized those numbers.

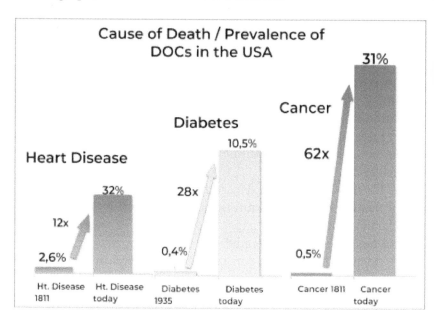

As you can see, heart disease as the cause of death rose 12 times, from 2,6% to 32%

The prevalence of type 2 diabetes went from 0,4% to 10,5%, a 28x increase.

And the worst disease of them all: Cancer! Death by cancer increased from 0,5% to 31% - a truly staggering increase of **62 times!**

But, I got to tell you: The usual suspects are not responsible for those rising disease rates!

It's obviously not about our genetics! It's also not about calories or too little exercise. It's not even about sugar or fructose or... insulin.

Yeah, you heard me right, ladies and gentleman - it is not about insulin!

So, what is it?

Let's take a quick look at the case of heart disease.

The mainstream explanation for heart disease is that

- We eat too much saturated fat
- This saturated fat contains cholesterol
- The cholesterol clogs our arteries, which researchers call "atheroslerosis", and
- Then we get a heart attack because of insufficient bloodflow to the heart

This chain of events also works for strokes.

This theory was popularized back in the 1960s by the scientist **Ancel Keys. That's** him as a young man... and here he is on the cover of Time Magazine. Quite a famous scientist, back in the day.

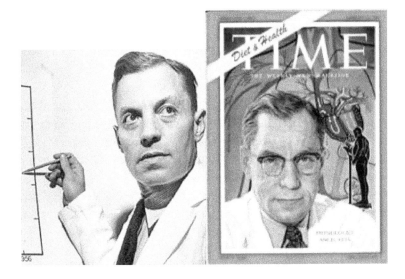

He tried to prove this theory by a study that looked at the correlation between nutritional cholesterol and deaths by a heart attack.

This study, the so called **"6 Countrys Study"** was more or less the very first earthquake of nutrition science - because it was the first one that connected our choice of foods to a deadly disease.

Here is his data from 1953:

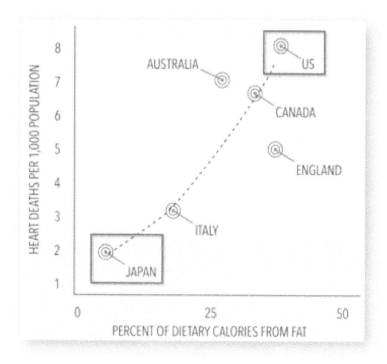

As you can see, Japan was the country with the best numbers:

At the time of the study, the Japanese people ate the least amount of fat. Only about 5 percent of their calories came from fat.

They also had the lowest rate of heart disease deaths: Only about 2 per 1000 people died of heart disease.

On the contrary – and on top of the chart – is the United States:

Those fat-loving younkees... they ate about 35 % of their calories from fats. Consequently, about 8 of 1000 people died of a heart attack. That is **4 times** the rate of Japan!

Ancel Keys stated that the high fat percentage, the high cholesterol intake was clearly the cause of all those heart disease deaths.

A lot of studies were done, which all wanted so show that this connection really does exists - although he didn't really have a biochemical mechanism how this should work.

So, did those studies show what Mister Keys wanted to prove? **No!**

In the best controlled studies that were done, the correlation was *inverse:*
The more saturated fat, meaning animal fat was eaten, the *less* people died! But these data were oftentimes not published or only years after the end of the study.

Nowadays, the correlation of cholesterol from diet and mortality goes like this:

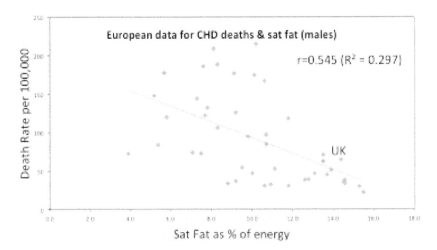

This is the real, unbiased data from the WHO themselves. Zoe Harcombe did this analysis, that's why the UK is highlighted.

The interpretation goes like in the chart from Ancel Keys:

On the x achsis, you see the percent of saturated fat of total energy. On the y achsis, you see the death rate for CVD, meaning cardiovascular disease.

And what does the red line tell us? Overall, the trend goes.... down! Down and not up! Meaning, the MORE people eat saturated fat, the less they die of a heart attack.

Here's the data for the women:

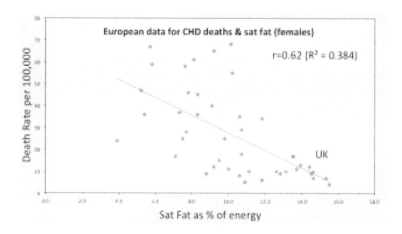

It's exactly the same thing: The correlation is even a little more pronounced than in men. So: Don't be afraid of animal fats. You know that meat won't hurt you... we've been eating meat for hundreds of thousands of years! It's in our genes!

So, did or does the mainstream explanation of heart disease hold true? Is it the cholesterol, the saturated fat? Nope, noparonimo!

But WHAT about Ancel Keys' super awesome 6 countries study? In that one, the correlation was quite convincing, wasn't it?

Well... turns out: If he had taken all the data that was available at the time, namely 22 countries, the graph would have looked like this:

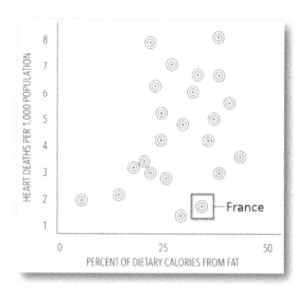

Correlation? There is none!

But: Who the heck are those guys, eating about 30% of their calories in fat... and still having very few heart attacks? Cest' la France, Monsiours et Madame, c'est la France!

Yes, the French like their fatty cuisine a lot – that's why this phenomenon was, and still is, called the **"French Paradox"**!

Well, it's not paradox at all, if you know that cholesterol is not the cause of this stuff.

All in all, there is no correlation, whatsoever! Mister Ancel maybe was... high as a kite when he was choosing the countrys.

Now, what is the real cause of atherosclerosis? You guessed it: Too much Omega 6.

Because oxidized LDL – LDL being the cholesterol - is the first step in atherosclerosis. And as Omega 6 fats oxidize the LDL-Cholesterol in our arteries, the Omega 6 fats are the cause of atherosclerotic plaques in the first place!

TUCKER GOODRICH:
"Turns out, that oxizdized LDL and, therefore, the oxidation of n-6 fats is essential to the initiation of atherosclerosis."

Now you know, who the real villain is: **Omega 6!**

You don't want to die of a heart attack? You also don't want your arteries to clog up? Then stop eating them!

But obviously: First you have to know where all of your Omega 6 is coming from! That's what we're going to talk about next: Our current Omega 6 Consumption.

Chapter 3:
Our current Omega 6 consumption

So, where do we get all that poisonous PUFAs from? This graph shows the percentage that the particular food group is contributing to our Omega 6 intake:

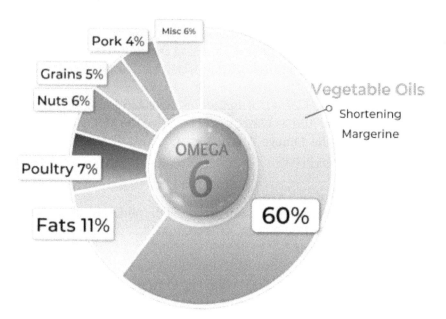

As you may have suspected, **vegetable oils contribute by far the biggest part with 60%.** Followed by fats with 11%.

Then, as you can see, also poultry has a fair share: 7 percent of all the Omega 6 fats come from chicken and turkey. This may surprise you as poultry is, after all, an animal source. So is pork, which also does contribute 4%.

But: We will talk about *animal sources of Omega 6* later on.

Last but not least in this chart, we have the Omega 6 coming from nuts and grains. Those also make up about 11%.

What's not in this chart is: Dairy, eggs, and beef.

These food groups are under "miscellaneous" - and those contribute between 1 and 2% of Omega 6.

Furthermore, the following foodgroups contribute each **less than 1 percent** of our consumption: All fruits and all vegetables. Nice, right?

To make this a little bit more practical for you:
In this table, we have an example of how these foodgroups are actually packaged as a dish – because people don't really eat or slurp their seed oils directly, we rather consume them as a meal ingredient.

Rank	Food Item	Contribu.(%)
1	Chicken & Chicken dishes	9.3
2	Grain-based desserts	7.5
3	Salad dressing	7.4
4	Potato / other chips	6.9
5	Nuts / Seeds & Nuts / Seeds dishes	6.5
6	Pizza	5.3
7	Yeast breads	4.5
8	Fried white potatos	3.5
9	Pasta & Pasta dishes	3.5
10	Mexican dishes	3.3
11	Mayonnaise	3.1

So, what dishes have is the most Omega 6 in it? What is to avoid, if we want to elimininate those fats?
Avoid everything that has a big portion of it directly as seed oils.
Mayonaisse has plenty of Omega 6, that's pretty obvious. Also salad dressing has a whole lot of seed oils in it. That should not be all that surprising, as it's kind of liquidy and greasy.
In general, you should be able to identify those sources pretty easily.

Then: Avoid everything that is fried – because the frying oils are **almost always from vegetable oils.** That's the reason why chicken and chicken dishes are number 1 on the list!

The same goes for potato chips and, of course, french fries.

Next on the list: The wheat flour, grain based desserts and dishes. What this means is more or less: Doughnuts and other sweet flour-dishes of that kind. Also: Non sweet dough-based dish like *classic pizza.*

In general: In all of those dishes that use some kind of dough, seed oils are added. And yeah, also wheat itself, the wheat flour, has Omega 6 in it.

Then, nuts: Those are probably self explanatory. Nuts are very fatty and their fat contains a huge amount of Omega 6 fatty acids.

Maybe you've asked yourself: "Why are pasta dishes also in this list? Is it really because of the wheat?"

Well, a little bit. But that's not really the major issue.

The major issue with these dishes, similarly to the Mexican dishes on the list, is,

1) The sauce that comes along with it! And

2) The chicken- and pork meat that comes along with the dish

Let's take Spaghetti Bolognese as an example. This dish has traditionally a tomato based sauce. So this one is fine.

With a classic bolognese dish, the issue is not with the sauce – it's the fatty meatballs, as we will see later.

Okay. Now that you know where all those nasty veggie Omega 6s are hidden, we should take a very close look at those vegetable oils themselves.

So: How much of the oils are actually Omega 6 PUFAs?

The chart I'm going to show you consists of the 8 top sold vegetable oils in the US. I arranged them in ascending order of their Omega 6 content. More specifically, their linoleic acid content.

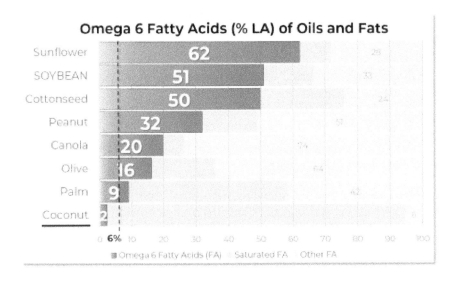

Omega 6 Fatty Acids (% LA) of Oils and Fats

The first group is the **superhigh Omega 6 group:**

Sunflower, soybean and cottonseed oil. They range between 62 and 50% Omega 6. That means that of a 100 grams of oil, 62%, meaning 62 grams are actually linoleic acid!

Then, we have the **high** Omega 6 group: Peanutoil and canola oil. These may no be that high, but they still have much. Too much!

Next up is the **moderate** Omega 6 group: Olive oil and Palm oil. If you really, really have to use an oil that's liquid at room temperature - for example for your salad - you could use those.

Unfortunately, there is a great bandwith of the Omega 6 content of olive oil. It can range *from 3% up to 25%!* So buy only olive oil, that has the PUFA content explicitly on the label. You should really stay below 10% Omega 6, maybe even below 6%.

As a rule of thumb, you should not really eat anything that has above 6% of its fats as Omega 6 fatty acids.

Then, we got good ol'd coconut oil: **Only 2%** of coconut oil is linoleic acid. Two percent!

That means that coconut oil is the best oil / fat to cook with! Coconut oil is the clear winner here. Use it plentyfully and prefer it over any other oil on this list.

When you take a look at this chart, what could you change in your nutrition to get rid of all those high and superhigh Omega 6 oils?

Yes, it is possible to change your cooking oil. Let's say, to coconut oil. Okay. But what about foods that you don't cook yourself?

Probaby, getting rid of all those superhigh Omega 6 oils is only possible by *avoiding processed foods completely,* isn't it? You're on the right track!

Okay, let's summarize what we've learned so far. Let's see what foods we should avoid.

Of course:
- Avoid vegetable oils directly. Don't cook with them, don't put them in your salad.

Then, as we've said in the slide with the dishes:
- Avoid everything that contains a huge portion of seed oils. Mayonaisse for example and fatty sauces in general. Dressing has lots of Omega 6s as well.
- Avoid everyting that is fried. Because 99,99% of the time, a seed oil is used for the frying. This affects all of your fried chicken products, french fries and the like.
- Avoid seed oils in processed foods. You can spot it on the label: If there's some seed oil in there, don't buy it.

Unfortunately, this stuff is in pretty much everything, I'm afraid. So don't think with your stomach.

Very important, not only within the processd foods category, but also at restaurants:
- Avoid dishes, that are based on some kind of flour dough. The oil used to make the dough, the meal, more palatable, is almost always a vegetable oil!

In the US, that is first and foremost soybean oil. Here's where your classic pizza and doughnuts come into play.

And last, but not least:
- Avoid all nuts - even a handfull is too much, as you will see later.

Regarding cooking - in the worst case, when you are cooking at home:

Choose palmoil or a low PUFA oilve oil for cooking. Or, even better: *Choose coconut oil!* Don't be afraid of the high saturated fat content., it won't harm you.

Let's change our point of view: It is probably easier to tell you what you can eat, right?

Summary of the RockSolid Diet V1

You can eat lots of *fruit.* And you can have plenty of *vegetables.* Do it. As long as they are low fat - which are pretty much all veggies and fruit - you can have those as much as you want.

As you may have figured out 'till now, the RockSolid Diet is *not necessarily a low-carb diet!* Carbs per se are not our enemies.

Yeah, I know. Carbs have quite a bad reputation these days because of... insulin! But in RockSolid Diet land, you can have them.

Accordingly, you can also have **classic carb sources.** But try to stay with the low fat ones, like rice and potatos.

Then, you can have **dairy:** Everything from fatty cheeses to milk to butter. Yes. Go for it.

And finally: You can have **meat, fish and eggs.** Those contain, after all, fatty acids from animal sources. So those are safe.

Or.... are they?

Well, let's take a closer look at animal fats. Maybe animal fats are not as healthy as we thought!

Now, regarding the Omega 6 content of animal fats, you will oftentimes find charts on the internet like this one:

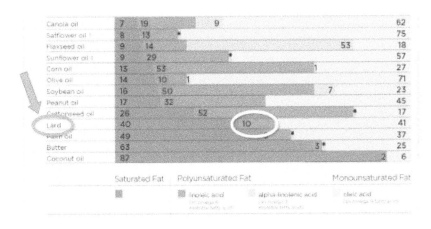

Here, we have pork fat, lard, as an animal fat source. And it shows that 10% of the fats is Omega 6. And we also have butter, with 3 percent. Butter has the same Omega 6 content as beef fat in general. Beef fat is also called tallow.

Ok, let's add those 3 values:

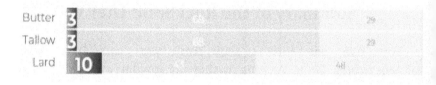

Butter	3	64	29
Tallow	3	66	29
Lard	10	42	48

However: Is this data really valid? Are these the values we're looking for?

No... they're not! There is a dirty little secret regarding animal fats...

Chapter 4:
The Animal Fat Anomaly

As you may have heard Dr. Knobbe say: Humans can not metabolize those PUFAs.

DR. CHRIS KNOBBE:
"We can't burn these for fuel properly. They're meant to be stored and used as signaling- and structural molecules, particularly in the mitochondria. They're not meant to be burned as fuel! That's why we accumulate these.

They accumulate in your cells and in your mitochondria. And this is where they wreak havoc! Because: It's polyunsaturated, and they're the ones that oxidize!"

Again: The Omega 6s just accumulate in our tissue... and then, they oxidize and oxidize.

Humans are mammals – and: We can't metabolize these fatty acids, these PUFAs. Guess what? Pigs can't do it as well!

So: As the production of soybeans has gone up dramatically in the last years and decades, so has the share of soy and other high Omega 6 products in the feedstuff of our livestock.

Lard has 10% Omega 6? Well, that would be great! But this isn't the case anymore. We are past that... by far!

Back in the day, pigs got barley to eat, especially in Europe. But now in the US, pigs not only get a bunch of soy products as foodstuff, they also get plenty of corn.

They even get the leftovers from distilleries, so called DDGS - *Dried Distillers Grains.* And of course, this stuff is superhigh in linoleic acid, Omega 6 fats.

As a consequence, the fatty acid composition is a completely different one!

Just go the the *US Department of Agriculture's* own homepage and see it for yourself:

When you look for "Lard", you really do get that 10,2% of linoleic acid. Which is the 18 carbon -2 fatty acid you got to look for.

Yeah, so: Ten percent. Hm.

But... that was the data in 1979!!

If you instead look for „Pork Fat", you get the value from 2011:

When you interpret the data: You take a 100 gram chunk of pork fat and there is 66 grams of fat in it. Okay. Out of those 66 grams, 11.8 grams are linoleic acid – which amounts to a whopping **18 percent** - which is a 80% increase!

So, this is the current status of lard, of pork fat. Which also has been confirmed by a lot of recent studies:

In a study from 2013, the control group – I repeat, the CONTROL group - had 18,7%! And the DDGs Group, the group eating the leftovers from the distilleries, they had an astonishing 22,8% of their fat being linoleic acid.

In a different study from 2016, the researchers experimented with varying amounts of these distiller grains. And they were able to bring the Omega 6 content up to an impressive **27,6%**! That's way more, than even canola oil has!

But "What about piggys on pasture?", I hear you say. "Those most be awesome, right?"

Well, the lowest Omega 6 value in a pig ever, that I could find, was in a polish study: Those pigs had 8,6% linoleic acid in the fat of their muscle meat... although they were not fed on pasture.

In all other studies I found higher values, so there's a lot of variation. Even wild boar had 12 percent.

All I all, in my own research, I concluded that the **average pork fat,** from both lard and muscle meat, is probably **around 17%** Omega 6, linoleic acid.

Yes, it really seems kind of high – but this is the data we are going to use. It went from 10% in 1980 to 17% in 2020. A 70% increase!

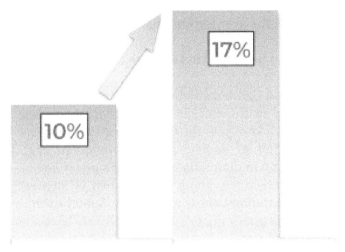

Pork Omega 6 1980   Pork Omega 6 2020

But what about everybody's favorite? Good ol' chicken!

'We love you so much' - as seen on the dishes chart. Does the chicken love us back? Not so much, unfortunately.

But with chicken, it's a different story than with pork. Chicken hated you right from the beginning! The Omega 6 value of chicken fat **was always superhigh.**

Here's what the USDA said **in 1979: 19,5% linoleic acid.** Again, canola oil level.

But, can't we bring that number up? Sure!

High 20% ranges are easily manageble if you give those sassy birdies a bunch of additional seed oils to eat, as clever scientiests have tried.

In one study, the researches really wanted to push the limits of time and space: The soybean group had 35% linoleic acid in the fat of the thighs. The record holders were the lucky chicks fed sunflower oil: *They reached mindblowing 38,5%!*

Now you see why fried fatty chicken products are just the very worst thing that you can eat, and why its contribution is the biggest of all foodgroups.

But what about pastured chicken? Meh, even pastured chickens reach 17% Omega 6.

In my humble opinion, looking at multilpe studies and the official data of the USDA, the **average Omega 6 percentage of chicken fat is around 22%.**
This is less than peanut oil but more than canola oil!

But... Ladies and Gentlemen, the real bummer is still to come:
Bad Omega 6s in the chicken turn over to their eggs, too. Of course! This is well known as the *Chicken and egg- problem.*
Eggyolks are full of linoleic acid: Conventional eggs have 15 percent of Omega 6 in their fatty acids. That's pretty bad...
"But hey", you're surely going to say, "then I'll just eat pasture raised eggs! Haha dummy, those are healthy. Superhealthy... right?!"
Won't work Amigo! Going full organic will only lower the Omega 6 percentage from 15 to...
What do you think? Five, 7, maybe 8 percent? Hm...
13,5 percent it is! Which is a negligible difference!
The eggs you think are super-awesome and super healthy... Yes, they are full of nutrients – and they're full of Omega 6s, too!
So, that's it? You can't eat any animal protein or fat because of its Omega 6 poisening? No my friend, it's not over yet. There may be some light at the end of the tunnel...
What about beef? What about steaks? And what about burgers? Fortunately, cows and **ruminants in general,** those have a special kind of bacteria in their gut, that lets them **convert the nasty Omega 6s to safe fatty acids.**
This means, that all meat from ruminants have very low linoleic acid values. Meaning, meat products from cows, lamb, sheep, goat and the like have around <u>2 to 4% of omega 6</u> – as well as their dairy products! Finally some good news I would say!
What? *Fish,* you ask? Well, fish has always *more* Omega 3 than Omega 6 in it – even the ones that are farmed. So don't worry about fish, just eat it as much as you want
Alrighty, let us put all these data back into the oil graph and see, what's really going on here:

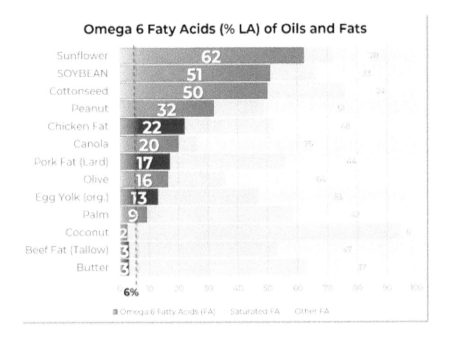

Omega 6 Faty Acids (% LA) of Oils and Fats

Sunflower	62
SOYBEAN	51
Cottonseed	50
Peanut	32
Chicken Fat	22
Canola	20
Pork Fat (Lard)	17
Olive	16
Egg Yolk (org.)	13
Palm	9
Coconut	2
Beef Fat (Tallow)	3
Butter	3

6%

■ Omega 6 Fatty Acids (FA)   Saturated FA   Other FA

As you can see, the blue bars: This is the *Animal Fat Anomaly* at its finest: Chicken, Pork and Eggs are now very bad food items and not really recommendable. Of course, it depends on how fatty the cut is.

Again, my advice: Avoid everything that's above 6% of Omega 6. *Which eliminates everything except coconut, tallow beef fat) and butter as fats for cooking and consumption.*

Now, that we've covered pretty much all animal protein and fat sources, let's go back...

You remember that summary? Well, that would have worked for the 1960s, before we started feeding our livestock crappy food, especially corn and soy. This means, we have to change summary of the RockSolid Diet. Quite a bit!

Yeah, I'm sorry.

Summary of the RockSolid Diet

Foods you can eat:
- **Fruits / Veggies / LF-Carbs**
- **Dairy**
- **Meat from ruminants, fish**

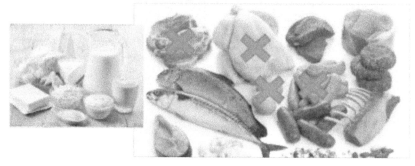

But: Now, with all this Omega 6 in animal fats floating around, you also have to **skip the following things:**

Meat from pork, meat from Chicken and eggs. Well, not a 100%. It still depends on the fat content.

Let's talk about how much Omega 6 we should / could consume. At the most!

[Chapter 5: See the Video for the calculations!!]

**You should / could eat a MAXIUMUM
of 10 grams of linoleic acid a day!**
This is the absolute upper limit, *10 grams a day.*

Now, with those 10 grams in mind, you should start to assess your very own Omega 6 intake. For example you could use our calculator at https://RockSolidDiet.com

Chapter 6:
The Omega 6 calculator - Introduction

Before we get into the spreadsheet, let's quickly try some nice, easy calculations, okay?

First of all: Omega 6 is still a fatty acid. So it's a fat. That means: If your food doesn't have any fat in it, then there can't be any Omega 6 in it, too.

Second of all: When there's plenty of fat in it, *then* the percentage of Omega 6 counts. To get to the actual Omega 6 amount, you just multiply the fat percentage times the Omega 6 percentage of that fat.

As we said above about fruits and veggies: Those are all very lean - so it does not really matter if the percentage of the Omega 6 within the food is high.

An apple, for example, has 0.2% of fat. *Of* that fat, 25 % is Omega 6 - which is pretty high, as you've seen with the seed oil graph. Comparable with canola oil.

However: As there is almost no fat in the apple, you won't get hardly any Omega 6 out of it! Even if the Omega 6 percentage is 25!

A big, 150 gram apple has 0.2% fat, which equals 0.3 grams of fat total. These 0.3 grams times the 25% of Omega 6 is 0,08 grams of Omega 6. **This tiny amount of Omega 6 is more or less representative of all fruits and veggies.**

Now, let's take some nuts, like peanuts. Okay, you're not going to eat 150 grams of peanuts, right? Maybe a 50 grams, a nice little snack. What is the fat content of Peanuts? Fifty percent. And the Omega 6 content? Thirtytwo percent.

So once more, we do a very simple multiplication: 50 grams x 50% of fat equals 25 grams of fat. Multiplied with 32% of Omega 6s, that is a nice and sweet 8 of Omega 6. Mmmm yummy!

Remember: We were shooting for a max of 10 grams a day... so we are already *almost at our limit,* with just this single snack of nuts!

And what about a couple of tablespoons of our beloved sunflower oil? Yeah, it's super duper healthy - for sure, that can't hurt that much, just 3 table spoons. Fifty grams.

Again, the calculation goes: 50 grams times 100% of fat – because oil is 100% fat - times 62% of Omega 6 equals **31 grams!**

Let's put this into perspective, let's put this next to each other:

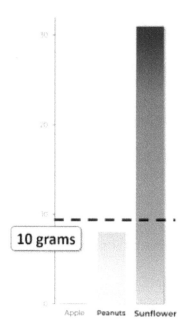

10 grams

Apple   Peanuts   Sunflower

Hm.... Yes... I would say: **This is a lot of Omega 6 from the oil!** Coming from 3 tablespoons of vegetable oil. Exceeding your absolute upper limit by a pretty 300%!

So, obviously: Avoid all seed oils in its pure form! That's the biggest chunk and the easiest one to avoid.

Alrighty, it's finally time for the calculator! Just go to my website https://RockSolidDiet.com

and download the thing! Be sure, to be logged into you Google account and then you can just get a copy of the calculator.

This copy then belongs to you - you can make all kinds of changes and tweaks – and you can also give it to your friends.

So go and get it! RockSolidDiet.com

(You should wach this part of the video yourself, because it shows you the calculator life in video. The part is in this video:

https://youtu.be/SUoqWbEntKc

And it starts at around minute 50.

Enjoy! And don't forget to then calculate your own foods

Acknowledgements
Thanks to the authors for their kind permission to publish these texts:

- **Dr. Thomas Seyfried,** Boston College

His website: https://tomseyfried.com/

His book at Amazon:
https://www.amazon.com/Cancer-Metabolic-Disease-Management-Prevention/dp/0470584920

- **Dr. Dominic D'Agostino**

His website: https://www.ketonutrition.org/

- **Travis Christofferson, M.S.**

His foundation to support Dr. Seyfrieds Research:
https://foundationformetaboliccancertherapies.com/

His books at Amazon:
https://www.amazon.com/Travis-Christofferson/e/B00OAOSZOA

- **Julie Foucher, M.D.**

Her website: https://pursuing-health.com/

_____

We also thank **CrossFit** for hosting the talks and their support!

Their website: https://www.crossfit.com/

Last, but not least: We would also like to thank **Robb Wolf** for his outstanding work and insightful platform,

His website: https://robbwolf.com/

THE
CARNIVORE DIET
OF
DR JORDAN PETERSON
& MIKHAILA PETERSON

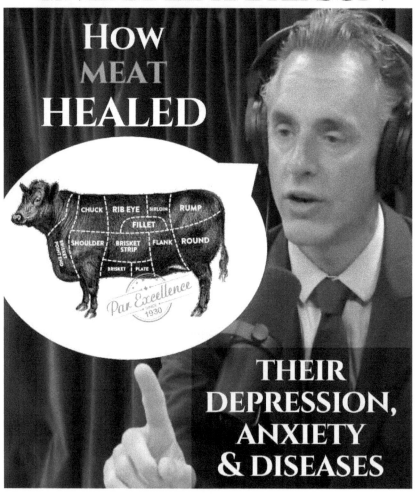

HOW
MEAT
HEALED

CHUCK | RIB EYE | SIRLOIN | RUMP
FILLET
SHOULDER | BRISKET STRIP | FLANK | ROUND
BRISKET | PLATE

Par Excellence
SINCE 1930

THEIR
DEPRESSION,
ANXIETY
& DISEASES

The book offers 11 Chapters of revised transcripts of Dr.

Jordan Peterson & Mikhaila Peterson on:

- how they cured their disease, depression and health issues with the carnivore diet and
- how ill people could start this kind of eating as well.

The Transcripts are as follows:
1. The Agenda with Steve Paikin Digesting Depression
2. Joe Rogan Podcast 1070
3. Joe Rogan Podcast 1139
4. Podcast Interview of Mikhaila Peterson with Robb Wolf, including blood work
5. Podcast Interview with Ivor Cummins
6. Talk by Mikhaila Peterson at the Carnivore Conference in Boulder, 2019
7. Mikhaila Petersons Blog: The Diet Introduction of her Lion Diet on YouTube
8. Mikhaila Peterson: Should you start an elimination diet?
9. Mikhaila Peterson: Jordan Peterson's Lion Diet
10 Mikhaila Peterson: The Lion Diet (Introduction of her diet on YouTube
11. Bonus-Transcript: Dr. Shawn Baker talking about his coronary calcium score and overall health status with years of being carnivore.

The transcriptions are revised, which means that the grammar and the wordsequences got corrected, adding phrases here and there, as well as leaving out other elements

Sources

Chapter

1)   Text (editors revised transcription) and slides based on   Youtube video:

Channel: „ CrossFit® "

Channel-Url:

https://www.youtube.com/channel/UCtcQ6TPwXAYgZ1Mcl3M1vng

Title: " Dr. Thomas Seyfried: Cancer as a Mitochondrial Metabolic Disease "

Video-Url: https://www.youtube.com/watch?v=KusaU2taxow

2)   Text (editors revised transcription) and slides based on   Youtube video:

Channel: „ CrossFit® "

Channel-Url:

https://www.youtube.com/channel/UCtcQ6TPwXAYgZ1Mcl3M1vng

Title: " Dr.   Dominic   D'Agostino: Emerging   Applications   of Nutritional Ketosis "

Video-Url: https://www.youtube.com/watch?v=_blupWpZ5F4

(Minute 32-43 / 54-57)

3)   Text (editors revised transcription) based on Youtube video:

Channel: „ Julie Foucher "

Channel-Url:

https://www.youtube.com/channel/UCWDto2R36n9pwwXq1HgjYHA

Title: " Challenging Conventional Cancer Care with Dr. Thomas   Seyfried - PH97 "

Video-Url: https://www.youtube.com/watch?v=_beGwmBYBlo

4) Text (editors revised transcription) based on Youtube video:

Channel: „ Anthony Chaffee MD "

Channel-Url:

https://www.youtube.com/@anthonychaffeemd

Title: " The Hard Facts about Cancer and Diet with Professor Thomas Seyfried of Boston College"

Video-Url: https://www.youtube.com/watch?v=1ebPZP9hBPA

5) Text (editors revised transcription) based on Youtube video:

Channel: „ Peter Attia MD"

Channel-Url:

https://www.youtube.com/@PeterAttiaMD

Title: " 30 – Thomas Seyfried, Ph.D.: Controversial discussion— cancer as a mitochondrial metabolic disease?"

Video-Url: https://www.youtube.com/watch?v=6PJfOFTaYow

6) **Article:** Taken from https://robbwolf.com/

Article URL:
https://robbwolf.com/2015/09/24/the-origin-and-future-of-the-ketogenic-diet-part-1/ (and following)

Article Title: „ The Origin (and future) of the Ketogenic   Diet "

Article authors: Dr. Dominic D'Agostino & Travis Christofferson

Milton Keynes UK
Ingram Content Group UK Ltd.
UKHW020633150524
442746UK00015B/507